REVIEWS

"Sharing our stories for the purpose of bringing glory to Jesus takes courage, strength, and so much vulnerability. From Claire's insights on the power that comes with taking control of our thoughts and the necessity of caring for our God-given bodies, to her willingness to dig into childhood trauma and her struggles with self-doubt in writing this book, she's shining a bright light on the God who heals, changes, restores, provides, and saves!"
—Liz Bruckner, writer and editor

"The first time I met Claire (via video call), she was not dancing. Instead, I saw a wounded young lady who was carrying a terrible weight of mental and emotional pain due to past trauma. As she shared her story with me over the following weeks, I had a sense that God wanted to do something special within her, and that if she was willing, God could take the 'mess' of her life and turn it into a 'message' of hope and healing.

The first time I got to meet Claire in person, she greeted me with a smile that lit up her entire face. There was a bounce in her step, and there were tears of gratitude in her eyes. God had done a miraculous healing within her!

To those reading this story, just know that what God did (and continues to do) for Claire, He wants to do for you as well. Healing is a journey, and depending on your starting point, it might be a long journey. But if you will do your part of sorting through your painful past, God will do the rest and bring a transformation to your mind and emotions that you never dreamed possible. So I challenge

you to dig your dancing shoes out from the back of the closet, dust them off, and try them on again. I bet you they still fit. And I know beyond a shadow of a doubt that you, too, can get to the place where you can dance it out every single day."
—Crystal Wallace, bachelor of Christian counseling

"Did you ever wonder what the 'Christian Faith' is supposed to do for you? It may be different than what you think. In 'Perpetual Healing,' Claire Cardinal pulls back the curtain to reveal the darkest corners of her soul. She's on a journey not for the faint of heart, and has no intention of playing the short game. Buckle up, this is about to get interesting, but who knows? You just might emerge from this, 'dancing it out every single day."
—Pastor Dwayne McCarty

"In her book, *Perpetual Healing: Dance it out Every Single Day*, Claire Cardinal shares her lessons for daily healing with honesty and vulnerability. She masterfully weaves stories and examples from her lived experience with lessons from the Word of God, providing the reader with real life strategies that are rooted in Biblical principles. If you're struggling and trying to strike a balance between your life as a believer in Christ and your physical or mental health challenges, this book will enlighten, empower, and encourage you!
—Julie A. Christiansen, author and psychotherapist

"Thought-provoking and raw, this book is real. Claire not only shares her personal experiences but really gets into the word and beauty of who God has called us to be—who he has made us to be. The three parts in this book go hand in hand and are necessary in becoming an overcomers. I highly recommend this sensitively written and well-researched book for anyone. Thank you for sharing your soul, Bean. You are an inspiration and so is this book."
—Shaila Stoddart

PERPETUAL
Healing

DANCE IT OUT EVERY SINGLE DAY

CLAIRE CARDINAL

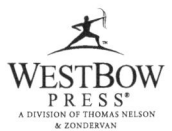

WESTBOW
PRESS®
A DIVISION OF THOMAS NELSON
& ZONDERVAN

WestBow Press books may be ordered through booksellers or by contacting:

WestBow Press
A Division of Thomas Nelson & Zondervan
1663 Liberty Drive
Bloomington, IN 47403
www.westbowpress.com
844-714-3454

Scripture taken from the King James Version of the Bible.

ISBN: 978-1-6642-8770-9 (sc)
ISBN: 978-1-6642-8771-6 (hc)
ISBN: 978-1-6642-8769-3 (e)

Library of Congress Control Number: 2022923800

Print information available on the last page.

WestBow Press rev. date: 1/6/2023

CONTENTS

FOREWORD

Claire and I have known each other for several years and have connected through genuine and relatable moments. As a working mother with my own practice as a faith-based counselor, I believe balance in life is important, especially when juggling life responsibilities. Therefore, I often reflect through a mind, body, and spirit lens with my clients, in personal relationships, and within myself to find balance. This book is Claire's heart and personal testament to the benefits of gaining support in each of these areas.

Claire authentically shares the process of her journey through testimony and reveals her heart in a relatable and transparent way to enable the reader to reflect on their own journey. She fulfills the role of an encourager in her shared experiences and empowers readers to share all aspects of their own story. She further provides good insights that have enriched the mind, body, and soul through each individual chapter. It is a refreshing read to those who have ever wondered about their own journey as a Christian and grappled with their own faith journeys.

When reading this book, one can expect to receive scriptures, learn about other personal testimonies, and ponder thought-provoking questions to consider for their own internal processing. Also, an enjoyable highlight are the song suggestions from each chapter, that welcomes the reader to "dance it out" in their lives. Finally, this is a read that can be experienced on an ongoing basis as our lives continue to change. With each life changing event, whether big or small, a new dance can be established through the balance of mind, body, and soul on a continual basis.

Claire is an inspiration and the embodiment of a superwoman in the Lord! Her super powers are not based on her personal strength, but rather on her determination to live her life with boldness through openness, hope, and the pursuit of balance with Jesus at the centre of the mind, body and soul. This book is a creative manifestation of her God-given super powers through the ever-changing seasons of life.

Nashola Pryce, M.A., C.C.C.

ACKNOWLEDGMENTS

To my husband, my "person," the Aaron and Hur to my inner Moses, the one who always reminded me to fight through the waves when they were overwhelming and violently crashing all around me, you revealed to me that I too was worthy of great love for who I am, your "Belle."

My husband, my confidant, the one who always believes in me and my dreams, regardless of whether I believe I can, you see my strengths and forgive quickly. You radiate the love of Jesus. What a gift it has been to discover together the greatest love we freely receive in Jesus.

Last but certainly not least, to the one who created me, who constantly shows up, because of who He is, this book would not be possible without God believing that I was more than my mistakes and inadequacies. This was never about me or what I could do, write, or say. It's always been about God, what He's done, and what He will continue to do. The healing I find daily in Jesus was always meant to shine a light toward His greatness and to bring Him glory every day!

INTRODUCTION

Deep within the editing process of this book, I felt unsatisfied with the introduction. How was I going to convey what this book was about and share my heart with you? I knew that it was already in me, if only I could find the words that would do it justice. Then, on the weekend before handing in this manuscript, I had a panic attack one night—another gut-wrenching, gasping-for-air, chest-clenching attack! The next morning, my husband, Jon, graciously woke up early with our dog, who needed to be let out, so I could sleep in. My body, mind, and soul screamed that it needed rest, so as you can imagine, I was thankful for his help.

As I pulled my tired body out of bed, I felt defeated. Soon after, I wondered how I could write a book about healing but still be walking through my own struggles. But, of course, the gentle voice of God whispered truth into my soul. That was exactly why I was writing this book because this is a daily healing. Perhaps I was sent a reminder about the true essence of my book. The message I'm sharing is about being healed daily in God, regardless of the darkness we may walk through. My ability to speak on this is magnified because of what I have gone through and still go through. He heals me daily.

Perpetual healing is the act of daily healing given to us by the great I AM, God, Jesus, the Alpha and the Omega. This book is for anyone who has suffered in the mind, body, or soul in their lifetimes. I'm here to break the commonly held idea that once Jesus heals you, the struggle is over and that your days should be filled with sunshine, unicorns, and rainbows; to break the pretense that if He really healed you, you shouldn't still be struggling; to help break the chains and negative thoughts that run through your mind, the thoughts that keep you from living your full potential in Christ and claiming the healing that He wants you to have and keep. This book was written for anyone who believes they are not worthy or that healing is not in the cards for them.

I've been filled with an undeniable healing in Jesus after years of fighting the waves that attempted to drown me. Through this, I have developed a simple principle that this book will address, broken into three parts: mind, body, soul. I would like to share the principle that the mind, body, and soul all need to be nourished for success. These three integral parts require balance for true fulfillment. At the center of it all is the heart, which should be Jesus, our guiding post and light in all things. Jesus at the center recognizes that our source of daily power and strength stems directly from Him. From there, we are able to radiate His love outward into every area of our lives and to those around us.

As I've mentioned, we have developed this idea that once Jesus heals us, there should be no more struggle. This could not be farther from the truth, in my humble opinion. Can Jesus heal you in the body? Can He heal depression, anxiety, or whatever mental struggle you are going through? Yes, He can! There is just one itty-bitty piece of information that you shouldn't forget while on your journey to healing. Your mind and body constantly adapt to your circumstances. Life changes; horrible events occur all the time. Life will shake you to your core, affecting your very being. Loss, grief, pain, hurt, struggle, or trauma will continue to present itself in your life. Your healing does not mean that you will never suffer again; in fact, Jesus never promised that.

John 16:33 says:

> These things I have spoken unto you, that in me ye might have peace. In the world ye shall have tribulation. But be of good cheer; I have overcome the world.

We are to find our peace in God who will help us overcome our trials and battles. This scripture brings hope. Imagine not having a loving God to lean on while going through unfathomable things in this world. Whether or not we believe in God, tribulations will occur, but because of Him, we have this undeniable strength. If we are not careful, our minds will control our thoughts and even actions. Furthermore, our minds will affect the state of our bodies and souls. What a wild concept, don't you think? How is it that our own minds can control our thoughts, emotions, and actions without our even realizing it? Healing of the mind is work and is a lifelong process.

I've written this book to share this concept with you. Perhaps healing from Jesus is the ability and strength to use the tools (or weapons) to fight back. The enemy would love nothing more than for you to hand over your mind, body, and soul in defeat. What a powerful tool for him to have in his hands. Why? Your actions begin in the mind; you first think before executing. That being said, if you allow your mind to run wild with negative, self-condemning, and evil thoughts, you cannot expect to produce good things. All three elements are interconnected, affecting one another daily. If the enemy can control that, then he will stop you from living the life that Jesus has for you.

We will learn how our bodies should be treated to benefit us. God can and will continue to heal our minds, bodies, and souls. To get the best outcome from the "warranty" that He has given us freely, we have a part to play in our daily healing.

The perpetual state of worship and praise is one of the greatest tools we have. One of my favorite ways to praise Him is through song. The act of opening our mouths to physically praise and worship, cry out to Him, or weep in His presence has a profound effect on all three elements of our beings. This is why within each chapter, you will find a song that, hopefully, will help you to enter into His presence.

As I've mentioned, I've divided this book into three parts: mind, body, and soul. Within each part are chapters that speak to the tools we need to conquer these concepts. I am not a certified psychologist, psychiatrist, or counselor. You might be wondering why you should read this book—*What can she help me with?* What I offer is a lifetime of knowledge, through trial and error, and wisdom from a God who has been so good to me.

Through the experience of peeling my sobbing body off a bathroom floor to get up and take care of my kids, I have learned how to pick myself up. Don't just trust my human experience; read on to learn what Jesus has taught me and how He has healed me, given me tools, and worked in my life in ways I never dreamed were possible. Do not misunderstand me; seeking counsel is important. I have sought that kind of help. There was definitely a time and place for it in my life, and my counselor helped me tremendously.

Simply, you can't do it without God's help. Trust me; I've tried many times. This did not happen overnight. Unfortunately, I lived through much heartache before getting to where I am today. At times, I have thought, *Why did He put me through this? Why did He allow me to live all these gut-wrenching experiences?* Most often, deep pain will reap deep growth in your life, should you choose to fight back. If I hadn't had the strength to walk through the test, where would my testimony be? The testimony is in the test; what we do with it is our choice.

At the end of each chapter, you'll find a list of questions and suggestions for you to answer. I've incorporated these questions to help you on this journey to healing. I pray that you would feel free to answer these questions honestly, and share your whole heart with God.

Before I share my heart and soul with you, why don't you listen to the song "Nobody" by Casting Crowns?

Never in a million years would I have believed that I would write a book. But as the above song expresses. Essentially I'm just nobody, attempting to share with everybody, about a God that has graciously saved my soul.

That is what this book is really about; it's about bringing Him glory through sharing my story. My prayer is that as you read this book, instead of seeing me, you would see God and His goodness.

PART I
MIND

Friend or foe, the decision remains in your hands. Daily training and sharpening of this entity are essential to win your battle.

1

GIRD YOUR MIND

What is the mind? A common definition is the element of a person that enables them to be aware of the world and their experiences, to think and to feel; the faculty of consciousness and thought.

The mind is one of our most powerful tools. It can make or break our success in all we do or try to accomplish. This is why we begin with this element of healing. While on this earth, our minds dictate all our decisions and actions; in short, the mind is our major control center.

Before you get up in the morning, you need to activate the mind, telling yourself to get out of bed. All of your actions start in the mind, and you do not complete any task without thinking about it. Perhaps you acted without thinking; the mind is still in control, even if you are not. The idea of your mind being in control without your consent is a common problem.

Why? So many of us simply walk, talk, act, and feel without thinking about it. Therefore, we have given our minds consent to conduct themselves in this way, even though we know better. Do we do this on purpose? The majority of us, I would say, don't purposely sabotage our thoughts. Similar to an abusive relationship, we have no idea how to put a stop to it, or perhaps we are blind to the abuse altogether. We may have struggled so long with self-condemning, negative, hateful, and abusive thoughts that we are numb to them.

The practice of learning to control our minds starts at a very young age. We either learn to control our minds, or we have no experience with the concept. This is why I am on my children like white on rice about their thoughts and mental states. See, if we are not taught to control our minds, then we don't know any other way. Time and hard work go into a mind that has the ability to control its thoughts and emotions. This does not come naturally. With four kids at home, I can attest to seeing firsthand which way the mind naturally gravitates. Instead of positivity, I've heard my children say things like:

"I can't do it."

"They are better than me."

"Why try?"

"I'm going to fail."

And the list goes on. My job as a parent is to tell them otherwise and to teach them about controlling their minds—to make sure they constantly think about what they allow in their minds. Proverbs 16:24 tells us, "Pleasant words are as an honeycomb, sweet to the soul, and health to the bones." You might be sweet and kind to others, but what you say to yourself, in private, is key to a healthy mind and soul.

Not only should we focus on what we allow in our minds but also what we remember. Life is filled with good and bad memories, as no life is perfect. Our experiences and memories directly affect our mindsets. This is why there is so much *circumstantial depression and anxiety*, which means that a person can experience depression or anxiety because of a certain event in his or her life. For example, postpartum depression is directly linked to that mother having had a baby. When I get anxious in life, there generally is a reason for it, whether an event is coming up or I'm nervous about a task to be accomplished. If we let it, it can snowball at us and become an avalanche, and we have no idea how we got to where we are.

2

As we age, it's natural for us to reminisce about our lives. Our memories are engraved in our psyches, but should we look back? That is a question in itself. If you are battling any type of mental struggle, one common tool is to focus on positive thoughts. Still, those negative, self-condemning, worry-filled, mind-controlling beliefs snake their way in.

The Bible story about Lot and his wife is a widely known lesson. Genesis 18–19 describes why they had to flee the city where they were living. The cities of Sodom and Gomorrah were very corrupt, with a whole bunch of sin happening right, left, and center. I wouldn't have wanted to hang around there, let alone call either my home. For context, I'll just tell you that God was very angry about the happenings in these cities. He decided that the only solution was to "clean up" (that is, eliminate) these cities. Hold on, though! God sent two angels to warn Lot to get out with his family before He destroyed the cities. Lot and his family were given simple instructions:

> And it came to pass, when they had brought them forth abroad, that he said, "Escape for thy life; look not behind thee, neither stay thou in all the plain; escape to the mountain, lest thou be consumed. " (Genesis 19:17)

Not complicated at all; basically, run, don't stop, don't look back! Because there are times when God does not want us to look back.

I propose that you start the practice of *mental amnesia.* Perhaps your circumstances have impaired your ability to look back on the works of the Lord. Practicing mental amnesia is imperative if you are going to fight properly against thoughts created to neutralize you as a child of God. Do this practice every day, until it's so natural that you don't realize that you're doing it all day. Don't be fooled or let your guard down, though, because as soon as you do, the enemy crawls in like a bat in the day. Did you know that bats usually look for solace during the day? These little creatures need a hole only about the size of a nickel to get into your space! They seek to roost during the day and live their best lives at night. We see them as creatures of the night, mostly because, well, they are creepy (sorry, I have no better word for it). But when you least expect it, they look for a place to set up camp, and they will come back all the time. In fact, during the winter, they usually hibernate for six months or longer. Take a minute to think about that. Do you want that creepy-crawly hibernating in your "attic," ever so quietly disturbing your peace? Close up any tiny holes, cracks, or leaks.

We need to solidify the foundation on which our minds are set. My family lives in a century-old home. The foundation is made of solid brick but still extremely old. Every spring, my husband goes around resealing any holes created from the wear of winter. We want to keep those creepy-crawlies out of our "homes," and that requires us to be vigilant with the nooks and crannies of our minds. Those little spaces that we don't close up will grow wider, and soon we will be mentally overwhelmed.

Trying to control our minds while in battle with our negative thoughts is utterly exhausting. Not only are we trying to push in positive thoughts, but we are fighting off the enemy on all fronts. When we are at war, the most successful side will be the one that has its soldiers on the front lines, prepared for battle. Rarely will the side that is caught off guard have victory over the enemy. The enemy is ready and waiting for us to take our minds off the prize.

We cannot control the circumstances of life—that is a difficult concept for most of us to accept. We think that if only we could control everything, then all would be good. What we can do, however, is control the way in which our minds react, a way that is conducive to a healthy mind, body, and soul.

As I traveled for the first time in three years since the start of the pandemic, there was so much anxiety in my mind. I tried to control what I could, but my mind was running at high speed, focusing on all the things that could go wrong. I knew that my mindset was wrong and that I needed to refocus on the works of the Lord.

A couple of days before boarding the plane to Victoria, British Columbia, God put a scripture on my heart:

> Finally, brethren, whatsoever things are true, whatsoever things are honest, whatsoever things are just, whatsoever things are pure, whatsoever things are lovely, whatsoever things are of good report; if there be any virtue, and if there be any praise, think on these things. (Philippians 4:8)

At first, I pondered why God had put this specific scripture on my heart, but then I realized He was speaking to my mind. This verse speaks to what we allow our minds to think on. I'm guilty of allowing my mind to see the what-ifs—and not in a good way. Jesus was telling me that it was time to start thinking about the now and what I know to be true, good, and praiseworthy. Do I know for sure that I will get sick? No, so that is not truth; that is fear (which is not of God). After thinking on this for a little while, I decided to build a mental picture. I imagined my sandals, the book I would read, my Bible, my sunglasses, and my favorite headband—an image I could hold while praising God and believing the good things He has promised me.

A big part of Philippians 4:8 speaks about trust. If we are going to think on things that are true, just, and pure (to name a few), then we need to trust that God's got our backs. It is not easy to do at times, but our job is to believe and trust in that. How can we claim that our trust is in Him while we fret over every little thing?

The peace that God can give us allows us to control our minds in a way that is impossible without Him.

> And the peace of God, which passeth all understanding, shall keep your hearts and your minds through Christ Jesus. (Philippians 4:7)

Trust me; I have tried to control my mind many times without Jesus being the center of my life. I always fail without Him. Life is not easy; it never was and never will be. An easy life was never promised. If you do not have God to lean on and to give you strength, then controlling your mind is impossible. Exactly as it says in Philippians 4:7, the peace He can give surpasses our own understanding. There is nothing like the peace that God can give us.

One of my favorite songs to listen to as I try to collect my thoughts and allow God to enter a situation is "Cover Me" by Mark Condon, which speaks to the peace of God:

> Cover me when I'm not strong,
> Cover me when I am going through the storm!

These lyrics are soothing to the soul when I'm trying to control the hurricane of thoughts and worries cycling through my mind. Ultimately, I ask God to be my shield and protector from the things that are affecting my mental state.

Again, we are not in control of our circumstances or what life throws at us, but with Him at the center, we are able to take hold of our minds and tell them which way to go.

I often think about Moses when I research the mind, as he had some major confidence issues. Moses was chosen by God to lead the children of Israel out of Egypt to the promised land. What an honor to be chosen to carry out such an important task, but he did not feel adequate. Most of us can understand how Moses felt; we get into our own heads. That was clearly a battle that Moses faced. His mind had convinced him that he was not up for the task. The enemy took his weakness and used it against him, and Moses chose to believe him. Read on a few scriptures farther, however, and you will find that God promised to be with Moses; more specifically, with his mouth. God basically assuring Moses that He would direct Moses in what to say and when to say it.

Later on, the Lord gets angry with Moses but tells him that his brother Aaron will take the task. This is an important point—God was angry with Moses. This was similar to parents who know their children can conquer a specific task, but the children choose to accept what their minds have told them. It's a mixed emotion of "Why won't you just listen to me?" and "Why are you allowing your thoughts to stop you from my purpose?"

> And Moses said unto the Lord, O my Lord, I am not eloquent, neither heretofore, nor since thou hast spoken unto thy servant: but I am slow of speech, and of a slow tongue. And the Lord said unto him, Who hath made man's mouth? or who maketh the dumb, or deaf, or the seeing, or the blind? have not I the Lord? Now therefore go, and I will be with thy mouth, and teach thee what thou shalt say. (Exodus 4:10–12)

The mind is a tool that requires sharpening and strengthening daily. A weak mind goes whichever way your emotional state is at that present moment. A strong and trained mind will control the thoughts that are allowed in and even what flows from the mouth.

The word *gird* is used many times in the Bible. Before I researched this particular word, it did not mean much to me. As I studied the Bible, however, I quickly learned that every word has a purpose. In fact, the first time I heard about the word *gird* in the Bible was during a counseling session. My counselor explained to me that I needed to apply the following to my life: "gird your loins." She explained what it meant to *gird your loins* in the biblical sense and why that was practiced. I was in awe with the meaning behind it; it made so much sense to me.

In the biblical era, men wore tunics. They were quite active, as men used their bodies in physical work much of the time. Wearing a tunic (similar to a dress) often got in the way when completing certain tasks. Can you imagine going into battle while wearing a tunic? So when it was time for battle, they tied a girdle around their waists and lifted the tunic between their legs, then used the girdle to tie it up securely. *Girding your loins* means preparing for battle; if you're going to fight properly, then you need to prepare properly for victory. You cannot have any loose ends getting in the way as you try to take the enemy; you must eliminate all potential distractions.

> Wherefore gird up the loins of your mind, be sober, and hope to the end for the grace that is to be brought unto you at the revelation of Jesus Christ; as obedient children, not fashioning yourselves according to the former lusts in your ignorance. (1 Peter 1:13–14)

The mind is a battle zone, and you need to gird your mind daily if you are to win. Put on your girdle, pick your tunic, gather any loose ends, and eliminate all distractions. If you do not gird your mind daily, the enemy will sneak in like a thief in the night, and you will not see it happen.

In fact, as I came to a coffee shop this evening to write, I had to put my girdle on. As a mom of four kids, with a busy house, messy house, and many other tasks I could be doing, thoughts of negativity flew every which way in my mind: *Why are you writing this book? You clearly do not have any time. You are a simple mom of four children. Who will care about what you think? There are so many authors more skilled than you. What makes you special? You can't do this. You will fail.* Yep, just as I'm attempting to write about girding your mind, I have to jump into battle myself.

Every day is a new day, filled with God's mercies and grace, but it is also a new day for us to slip and fall. Am I saying that we should never fall? Of course not. We are human, and the Lord knows that we will fall. But we need to stay sober and alert, watching for the enemy who would love to corner us without our girdles in hand! The truth is that we still will have thoughts that have no place in our minds, but the trick is to catch them as they are trying to creep in.

Controlling your mind is the foundation of a healthy mind, body, and soul. If you cannot control it, then the enemy constantly will steal the truth from you. When you fall repeatedly, it is extremely difficult to make any headway and receive what God has for us. As babies learn to walk, the first weeks consist of them constantly falling and not getting anywhere. But as they improve their balance and stop falling, there is progress. Soon, our babies are on the go. Then the challenge is to stop them from getting into everything.

Similar to a baby, we are to learn and train ourselves daily, remembering to gird our minds, thus resulting in less "falling." We can only receive what we believe is rightfully ours. If we do not believe that we are worthy of God's love, salvation, and power through the Holy Spirit, then we will not fully receive it. We will find ourselves playing a game of yo-yo with Him, consisting of God filling us with His love and spirit, but then we give it back because we don't feel worthy. The back and forth can continue until we tell our minds and the enemy what's what. We must claim it in our minds and hide it in our hearts.

You know where your major mind weaknesses lie (and if you don't, then you absolutely need to find out).

There are certainly a few that constantly bounce back from time to time in my mind—unworthy of love, weak, small, and unimportant. Then there are times that I get a punch in the gut out of left field, something that I've never battled with but is ever present. If my mind is not ready and girded, then that potentially can bring me to a place I have no business being.

Think on that: you have no business in the place of mental darkness and condemnation. Keep that door locked, and throw the key away.

Sunday mornings are usually busy as we get our four kids out the door for church, while I try to put myself together and not leave the house a complete disaster. My daughter is sure to yell from upstairs,

"I have nothing to wear." My ten-year-old might show up dressed but completely mismatched. Does he care? Not at all, so I usually know when to pick my battles.

One particular Sunday morning, while enjoying our coffee, my husband and I were looking at some old family photos. We sat there, reminiscing and laughing at how young and immature we looked. After that, it was time to hustle and get ready for church. As I stood there looking in the mirror, a spirit of unworthiness swept over me. I began to question whether I belonged in church. Thoughts of self-hate overwhelmed my soul. Some of them that tried to take over that morning were as follows:

Look at you. This is just a facade. You do not belong in church.
You haven't changed at all. You are unworthy of God's love.
You were not raised in church. What are you doing here?

I walked into our bedroom and looked at my husband. He looked in my eyes, and we both knew how the other was feeling—he was feeling exactly the same thing that I was going through. The heavy weight over both of us was undeniable that morning. The enemy tried to bring us to a place of self-condemnation through our pasts, but we saw it coming before it started to affect our minds. We knew that it was not the spirit of God working in us that morning; this was not the way He makes His children feel. There is no condemnation in Jesus. He does not dangle our past in our faces. If we hadn't had experience in girding our minds, I don't even like to entertain the thought of where we might be today.

It is important to note that we cannot blame all our battles on the enemy. There are times we give him too much credit. We allow certain things into our lives that affect our minds. What about that toxic relationship we keep going back to? Maybe we allow our minds to run while scrolling through social media?

Come on now; let's be honest. There is a handful of negative news on social media on any given day. If you don't practice mental amnesia, and you constantly think about negative events that occurred in your life, then you are not helping yourself.

When was the last time you prayed? How about your Bible—does it have dust on it? Who are your friends? Do they empower you? Do you take care of yourself, or are you an afterthought?

Matthew 6:21 tells us, "For where your treasure is, there will your heart be also." Your mind will follow your heart. If you fill your heart with God's treasure, controlling your mind will be much easier. Things that are from God are pure, true, good, and praiseworthy. Whatever you fill your time with and prioritize it, your mind and heart will follow.

I make time with God the highest priority in my life. On most mornings, I'm awake before my kids so I can read His Word and spend time in prayer. Putting the Lord first has allowed my heart size to triple for Him. Since I have done this, my heart yearns for more of Him and the Word. Controlling my mind and emotions is simple when my day surrounds Him in whatever way it can. Why? Because when I fill my day with the things of God constantly, my mind is focused on Him. My treasure is found in Him completely; thus, my heart and mind are right where they should be.

1. Can you identify the weak areas within your mind? What thoughts do you battle with most? List them here so you can begin to acknowledge them.

2. Find a scripture (or scriptures) that you can use to fight the battle in your mind. This will be specifically tailored to your personal battle.

3. What practice can you put into place today to begin the process of girding your loins (also known as girding your mind)?

4. Listen to the song "Cover me" by Mark Condon. Allow the peace of God to cover your mind today, and ask Him to help you find that peace in every storm.

2

LIFT YOUR HANDS

If you have ever experienced depression, then you know that it weighs you down entirely. It's a personal burden that you carry, often on your own, until you seek the right kind of help. Even then, you can feel completely alone, as if you are the only person in the world to ever feel this way. Not a soul on this earth can possibly understand how you feel, how you hurt, how you feel emotionally dried up, and how you keep on keeping on.

As I researched the definitions of *depression*, I quickly realized that none of them described what a person feels. Sure, the definitions were accurate, but they didn't feel accurate enough. The word depression makes me think of some sort of pressure applied, put on, or carried by a person. Obviously, that's not a dictionary definition, but having suffered through it myself, that's my description of it in my own words.

To be deep in depression is to feel a constant pressure on your mental, emotional, and physical well-being. It's a feeling that tells you to get up and accomplish your daily tasks, only to be struck down with a pressure telling you to keep lying there. Unless you have truly experienced depression, you cannot fully understand how a person feels, which makes it extremely difficult for you and other loved ones to support that person. If you haven't felt certain emotions, it can be hard for you to understand the person who is depressed. Empathy comes from a place of knowing, from the ability to feel what the person is going through.

Since the age of twelve, I have dealt with depression that comes and goes in waves. At times, I had no idea what was happening within me. I just knew that there was no motivation or happiness in me when there should have been. For years, I just kept going, with an acceptance that this was who I was. From meeting my husband to having children, I carried this weight with me wherever I went— waves of anger, sadness, complete hopelessness, no motivation, and unfulfillment. There were many times in my life that I found myself lying on the bathroom floor in tears, emptying all the emotions with which I was dealing. I believed that life would be better for everyone without me in it. I've experienced many of those moments—the ones I don't share with just anyone, as they hold shame. I'd lock the bathroom door and lie on the floor, unable to pull myself up and out and looking at a bottle of pills that could end its all. I had no self-worth. I believed that my life was not important and that if I was not around, my children and my husband would be better off. Obviously, I didn't follow through on these thoughts.

I peeled my sobbing body off the bathroom floor more times than I'd like to admit. The pressure to keep going was too much to bear at times. As it came in waves, I would be fine for a short period, riding a high from something that life had given me. Then, all of a sudden, something would switch in my mind, and I'd be back to the depressed, self-loathing me. The feeling of wanting to lie in my bed for days and do absolutely nothing would overcome me at the best of times. I didn't want to lie in bed so I could watch movies and binge on candies and chocolate. No, I was in a place of self-paralyzing torture, created by the depressing thoughts roaming through my mind.

Somewhere inside, it simply felt better to lie there and do nothing all day. My heart felt empty. My soul had a nonexistent sensation to it. How could anyone who had the feelings I had have a heart and soul worth fighting for?

Most of my life, I have felt small and weak; it's the emotion I've carried forever. Since my childhood, people have said, "She's so dainty [fragile, sensitive, weaker than most, small]." They probably didn't mean anything hurtful by those words, but the words shaped and formed me. After hearing those words over and over, they became deeply instilled in my psyche. I set so many limitations on myself because I believed that I just could *not* because of who I am. I made myself small and meaningless within my own mind.

If you have felt this way, then you know that it starts to chip away at you mentally. When you don't believe in yourself, it quickly turns into a deep depression. The thinking is, *Why try? It's not like I'm capable of much.* You tell yourself, "Be careful not to hurt yourself. Watch out so you don't overexert yourself—you know that your capabilities are limited."

Knowing what I know now, I realize things could have been great, if I'd had, flowing within me, the kind of spirit David had in his youth. You can find the story of David and Goliath in 1 Samuel 17. David was the youngest in his family, just a normal guy who tended to the sheep. While his brothers were at war with the Philistines, they needed someone who was capable enough to defeat Goliath. Somewhere in all of this, David showed up in the war zone with provisions and claimed that he could take down this big guy everyone was talking about.

David was not being arrogant or overconfident. He knew who was on his side, and that changed everything for him. David knew what kind of God he served, and he was filled with *God confidence*—a kind of confidence that can only be obtained when you know who your Creator is, and you fill your mind with His promises. David defeated Goliath with much ease because of the Lord. Know who you serve and who God calls you out to be!

The problem with depression is that the more you lie down, loathe, and allow yourself to sink, the deeper the hole you dig. I'm a firm believer in allowing yourself to have a day or two of *dolce far niente*, which is Italian for "pleasant relaxation in carefree idleness." But watch out when it becomes your norm; then, it is depression. The difference is that with *dolce far niente*, you have chosen to relax and be carefree; with depression, you have absolutely no drive to do anything.

I have experienced this, and it's a thin line that needs to be carried with great intentionality. You need some vacation time away from work, or you need some time away from the family to gather your thoughts and recharge. This is absolutely OK; everyone needs that! In fact, allowing yourself this time is crucial to your mental health and to keep a healthy mindset. When we push ourselves past our limits, then our mental health will start to spiral.

Growing up, I was taught to always have something on the go; there was always a household chore to be accomplished. You want rest? What? That is for the weak! Every day should be filled with many tasks. That is where you find your worth. Didn't you know that? *No!* That couldn't be more wrong.

Until a few years ago, I believed that I had failed if I didn't fill my time with chores and serving others. Do you know how exhausting it is to constantly be busy with a million things to make yourself feel worthy? This type of mental state is absolutely depressing and is such a vicious circle. If we don't prove our worth to ourselves and others, then we become depressed. When we do "prove" ourselves, we are exhausted, which leads to depression and then wondering what is wrong with ourselves.

Social media is the worst for this nowadays. Left, right, and center, we see posts about all the things that everyone else has accomplished that day. *Wow, look at her living room. It's perfection, and she baked cinnamon buns.* What we don't see are the screaming kids in the background or that she went right back to bed after posting that. It's depressing for us when we measure ourselves against unrealistic standards. Our worth is not measured by how clean our houses are or how well we bake. True worth is found in Jesus, when we understand that we are unworthy but through Him, we are made new. Then we will get to a place of constant praise over all the little things. We will thank Him for providing us with the strength to get our kids to school, to make supper, to clean the bathroom. Or we will praise Him because we were able to rest in His presence, and we will ask for strength to keep going. When we throw our hands up in the air, we will give and start our day with Him because only His strength is sufficient for us. We are OK with accomplishing whatever His will is for us today, even if it looks different from what we had planned.

As a young child, wife, and mom who has battled depression, I know firsthand how important it is to lift your hands. You want to give up, throw the towel in, walk with your head down, and lie in bed all day, but this is not how you will conquer your battle. It has taken me years to come to that realization. The heartbreak, trials, and emotional upset I've been through brought me to a place of desperation.

Before I reached that place, though, I had someone by my side. Everyone needs their "person." I met my husband, Jon, when I was seventeen. On our first date, there was no doubt in my mind that he was the one, and the feeling was mutual. As Luke said to Lorelai in *Gilmore Girls*, "I'm all in!"

Jon was a breath of fresh air after all the disasters I had dated. Together, we have been through so much that I could write a book on all our life's adventures. He was unaware of my personal battles when he met me, but not too long afterward, he saw what I was carrying. My mind does not comprehend why he stayed with me when he found out that I was battling depression—it could get pretty bad when I went through a tough time.

Writing this book has made me realize that Jon was sent to me by God Himself. Only the Lord knew that I would need Jon and that he would be a steady hand to lean on in my biggest trials. In my darkest times, lying on the bathroom floor or wanting to lie in bed for days, he was there. This man would hold me, pick me up, and be the voice of hope to get me through. The important part of his help was holding me up; he never let me stay down—with depression, this is crucial. Sure, he allowed me to have a day in bed, wallowing in self-loathing. He knew that I needed it, but he never let me stay there for too long. After a certain period, it was time to get up and do something, even if it was simply sitting on the couch, having a coffee.

Be alive and look alive because you are alive. Take baby steps toward getting you strong, where you need to be. When I lay on the floor in tears, telling him that he would be better off without me, it broke his heart. I looked into his eyes and saw the heartbreak, and sometimes, he seemed not to know where to go from there. It wasn't because he wanted to leave me, but he wondered how in the world he could make this better. Most times, he simply told me how much he loved me and how important I was to him. There were times when he got angry with me—how could I say such things?

This is a shout-out to anyone who has stuck by a loved one who is fighting depression. It's not easy, and the road is long. I see you, and you are more important than you can possibly realize. You have kept that person going.

Jon was my Aaron and my Hur on the mountaintop. In Exodus 17, you can read about the battle between the Amalekites and the Israelites. Joshua was sent out with some men to fight the Amalekites. Moses stayed on top of a hill with hands raised, and as long as he did that, the Israelites saw victory. If he lowered his hands, then they would begin to lose their battle. It was extremely important for Moses to keep his hands lifted. Naturally, he started to tire, but Aaron and Hur offered support by holding up Moses's hands!

God places people in our lives to help us when we grow tired and weary. We were never meant to go through this life alone. There are times when you will need help to hold up your hands, and perhaps you will do the same for someone else. At least lift your hands up, and keep them up. You're tired? You feel like you can't do this anymore? There is not a thing wrong with that, but you need to reach out for help. Allow someone to be your Aaron and Hur, just like my husband, Jon, has been to me.

> And it came to pass, when Moses held up his hand, that Israel prevailed: and when he let down his hand, Amalek prevailed. But Moses hands were heavy; and they took a stone, and put it under him, and he sat thereon; and Aaron and Hur stayed up his hands, the one on the one side, and the other on the other side; and his hands were steady until the going down of the sun. (Exodus 17:11–12)

You need to start—just begin somewhere—one day at a time. Lifting up your hands and keeping them up requires you to be intentional about it, and it takes time, along with strength. If you try to hold your hands up all day for the very first time, you will quickly become tired because you have no stamina.

When I speak to the act of lifting your hands, it is not only physical; in fact, performing the act in your mind is much more important. Each day, you need to lift your hands mentally. Look to the one who gives you strength and joy. To do this is the complete surrender of your mind; you are acknowledging that God controls all and will fill you with His joy. You need to find out what brings you down personally and work on those triggers daily. How should you work on them? You should lay these burdens at God's feet by lifting your hands and allowing Him to completely renew your mind. You have a part in this, and it is a daily act of healing of the mind. Your mind is a muscle that needs to be strengthened and conditioned daily.

Many of us need to arrive at a certain place before true healing can work inside our minds and souls. A few years back, I found myself in a place of deep desperation because of life's circumstances. When life happens, we often do not understand why these events occur. To this day, I do not fully comprehend why I've been dealt this hand, but I know that it can be used to help someone else who might be struggling. If we can use our hurt, pain, and desperation to help others, then it will be worth it.

Girls admire their fathers; they look to them for guidance and love. Most often, when choosing a husband, they unconsciously may choose someone similar to their fathers. It's not all the time, but if you were blessed with a good father, then you surely will want your husband to have similar qualities.

Girls also seek love and approval from their fathers. If they do not receive it at home, then they will seek it elsewhere—and most times in unhealthy ways. For years, I looked up to my dad, my papa. I constantly sought his approval. If I did something for which he could be proud, then I believed that was success. In my teenage years, Papa and I were extremely close, and I relied on him entirely. Fast-forward to later in life, when I was a married woman with children, living my own life, and making decisions that were best for my family. One day, I decided to follow Jesus, and I never looked back. Unfortunately, my father does not approve of my being a Christian. I believe he feels that he's been replaced, and even after several conversations, I haven't changed his thinking.

Hurtful words were said, but most important to me was that he made it clear that our relationship was over. Not being able to speak with him broke me. His not caring about how I'm doing or how my children are doing crushed my soul. To get to a place of acceptance took a long time, and I went into a very dark place. Why doesn't he care? He used to tell me how proud he was of me, and now he can't even talk to me. I did try to fix things—I tried until it nearly killed me and my family, emotionally. You see, when Mom is sinking, everyone else feels the effect. Lashing out at Jon was not rare in this dark time. I couldn't understand, and I was so angry that it had to be someone's fault. This was a serious depression, and I didn't know how to stop myself from falling into it.

Anger is a secondary emotion. In most cases, we usually feel another emotion first that we have yet to figure out or admit. After a while of torturing myself, I finally decided to speak with someone about the issue affecting my entire family. My counselor helped me see a groundbreaking idea—I needed to grieve the loss of my father. Although he was not dead, the relationship we once had was gone. My sole focus always had been on how I could fix this relationship. *When will Papa come back? Can I change myself enough for him to love me?*

My counselor also asked if I was willing to give up my relationship with Jesus for my father. She asked this because I told her that is what he wanted. My answer was a swift *no*. Nothing should come between that relationship. You can see where she was going with this, right? If I wasn't willing to give up what my father needed me to give up, then I would have to learn to let go. Once I understood that my anger stemmed from my hurt, pain, and grief, I could better manage those emotions.

No doubt the biggest help was realizing that it was time to grieve that relationship. Clearly, my trying to hold on to it was not helping anyone. In this time, I also found my life scripture, the one that I hold onto daily and that speaks to me in a way no other scripture does:

> Be still, and know that I am God, I will be exalted among the heathen, I will be exalted in the earth. (Psalms 46:10)

This spoke to me on such a profound level, as I constantly tried to control all the wrong things instead of simply being still and allowing God to be God. This scripture was like honey to my soul; it told me it was OK to be still. I was raised to constantly be busy to prove to everyone how worthy I am. Psalm 46:10 tells me to stop relying on what I can do and how I can fix things and to be still and allow God to work in my life.

Ecclesiastes 3 speaks to a time for everything and a season for every activity; in particular, a time to tear and a time to mend, a time to be silent and a time to speak. As much as it broke my heart, this was not a time to mend or a time to speak. Rather, I needed to be still and silent. I do not know if our relationship will ever be mended. Because of the grieving process, however, this thought bothers me less and less every day. I do know that I will always love my father, even if that means having to do it from a distance.

My broken relationship with my father brought me to a place of desperation. I had no idea how I was going to dig myself out of this one. Jon was at a complete loss; he had no idea how to help me. I felt no emotion except anger. At that time, I was teaching Sunday school, which was something I enjoyed doing, but on one particular Sunday, I just felt empty. Still, I managed to drag my body out of bed. As I walked over to the service with all our Sunday school kids, "big church" was just finishing up with an altar call. I stood at the back, close to the doors, watching as the kids joined their parents. I didn't want to go in and participate, but I contemplated what to do with the way I was feeling. I was extremely tired, emotionally, and annoyed that I still felt this way over someone who had moved on. I marched up to the altar, not knowing what I was going to say to God. I knew that I needed a healing, perhaps the biggest of my life. Depression had to leave me. I could not do this any longer on my own.

As my hands lifted up to the God I knew could completely heal me, I was speechless. I stood there and wept, simply stilling my mind, body, and soul. I handed over all of the hurt from my past to Him, asking that He take it and renew me. *Bam!* I know—so dramatic, but that's what it felt like. Something shifted in my mind and soul. I knew that God had healed me. I had a strong impression on my heart from God saying, *Finally! You have waited so long to come to me and hand it all over!*

In Luke 8:43–48, we learn about the woman with the issue of blood. She had lived with the disease for twelve years. What a long time to live with something like that. Certainly, she felt hopeless after having seen many doctors but with no healing for twelve whole years! I read these scriptures, and tears start to flow. I felt her heart, the desperation she must have felt within her soul. She knew that Jesus was passing through, and this was her chance to be healed. She knew it was time, if she could get to Him somehow. Filled with desperation and faith, she knew that if she could just touch the hem of His garment, she could experience healing. Jesus was so powerful that if she could just touch a piece of Him, that would be enough.

As I walked up to the altar that morning, something stirred in my soul, telling me, *All you need to do is move, and lift your hands up.* There was no strength left within me to cry out, but I was filled with enough desperation to move toward Jesus and simply get a touch from Him.

All you need to do is begin to lift your hands and give your whole heart to Jesus. Let Him do the rest. He wants to meet you where you are. Wherever that may be, He can meet you in any mental state. If you are thinking that you're too far gone, that is exactly where you need to be. Being in that place of desperation is the best place to be to receive what He wants to give you. Why? When you are desperate, you have no choice but to lay it all down at His feet. As you realize your strength is not sufficient, you start to rely on Him completely.

The song I feel that is fitting for this chapter is called, "Dawn" by Rebecca St. James. Listen to the entire song—it begins in a dark place and slowly moves to a place of desperation and healing. She sings about lifting your arms and receiving healing. The first time I heard this song, my heart wept, and I instantly connected to this song. I knew exactly what she was talking about. She sings about the promise from God—a new day coming, even in the darkness. In the darkest hour, we may feel that dawn will never come, but God brings a new day filled with new mercies and grace.

As you wake up every morning and see God's promise, you are given a new day to be filled with His daily healing, another chance to start over and to continue claiming your healing walk with Him, as He holds your hand or, at times, carries you.

1. What emotional triggers bring you to a place of depression or other mental struggle? If you haven't taken note of that, intentionally watch your emotions, and write down your emotional triggers.

2. What are you desperate for Jesus to heal in your life or within you? Find a quiet place today where you can go to talk to Jesus about it, and hand over your burdens to Him. Make sure to allow time for yourself to be still, and allow Him to speak to your heart.

3. Find your life scripture. This may take time. Read the Bible, ask God to speak to you, still yourself, and listen. You will know when you've found it. Write it down here. Why does it speak to you?

4. The song "Dawn" by Rebecca St. James opens my heart to newfound hope where there seems to be none. Play this song and accept the emotions that well up from inside you, and simply wait on the Lord.

3

YOUR SUNRISE

> For God hath not given us the spirit of fear; but of
> power, and of love, and of a sound mind.
> —2 Timothy 1:7

Second Timothy 1:7 tells us clearly that fear is not from God, that we are not filled with fear; instead, we are filled with power, love, and a sound mind. Fear can stop you dead in your tracks. Fear is a liar. The things that we fear usually have not happened yet, but we are afraid that they will. Fear is looking into the future—whether hours, days, or months—and predicting doom and gloom.

There are times when your fear is warranted; perhaps a certain event happened in your life that marked you. You were left a bit traumatized. Fear tells you that you are likely to experience some sort of discomfort or pain. Anxiety stems from fear—you are worried about something undesirable. Because you know, logically, that you can't predict the future, you should be able to kick fear to the curb. Unfortunately, it usually doesn't work that way, and that is a battle in itself.

The twelve-year-old version of me got overly excited about many things in life. Easter is coming? Well, you can bet that Claire is pretty jazzed and cannot contain her excitement. I would make myself sick—not willingly, but my emotions got the best of me. Whether it was a good event or an event that was unsettling, I would feel not quite well.

One summer, my sister and I were playing in my grandparents' living room. I was playing the piano, and she was standing on a stool, close to the brick fireplace. She kept bugging me about wanting a turn to play the piano. Of course, since I was older, I believed she should wait until I was done—and I was not planning on finishing for a while. Isn't that what siblings do to each other? They like to torture one another in any way possible.

My sister was getting antsy, jumping around, and climbing up and down on that stool. Suddenly, I looked over and saw that she had fallen, head first, on the brick fireplace. The whole family heard the screaming and came running in. My dad helped her up and examined her from the front, while I stood behind her and told them what had happened. Much to my surprise, I saw a very dark stain on the back of her pajamas and screamed, "She's bleeding!"

I laugh at my reaction now, but my parents were not happy about my screaming while they were trying to keep my sister calm. My parents ended up bringing her to the hospital to get stitches. I stayed home with my grandparents and tried to calm myself. Of course, I felt just horrible about her accident and probably felt it was my fault. That night when she got home, all was good, and there was nothing to worry about. Well, wouldn't you know it? I woke up sick that same night. It was only a few years ago that I put two and two together—my worry and anxiety had me sick; it was not something I had eaten.

Why didn't I see this pattern before? I have been sick so many times in my life, but we just chalked it up to something I ate. The first Christmas I spent with Jon's family, I was sick, but again, I believed that it was a bug or food-related. Without my being aware, my body reacted to milestones in my life. Our wedding day—by now, you can surely imagine how I felt that day. By the time we were to have our first dance, I was an empty shell. Jon held me up throughout the entire song because I was just drained from the emotions.

Clearly, worry and anxiety have attempted to get the best of me for longer than I have imagined. Life can throw curveballs, and all we can do is try our hardest to dodge them. The reality is that if we are not careful, the buildup of worry and anxiety will consume us.

There was a time in Jon's and my life, about ten years ago now, when we felt completely alone. We were far from home and had not come to God yet. We had two kids and one on the way, and we were moving to a northern community, where we had no support. We simply attempted to get through each day. Our move was not the smoothest, and although I knew that others had experienced this, I felt totally and utterly alone.

The second night in the hotel, before we were to make our way to our new home, I was hit with a stomach flu. I cringe just writing that term; if you've ever suffered through it, then you know its volatile nature. Far from home, with all our stuff packed away in a moving truck, I'd never felt so helpless. And remember—I was pregnant with our third at that time. That night, I was worried I might need to go to the hospital because I was dehydrated. Simply put, I was traumatized by this particular event.

Then we got to our new home, and the rest of the family fell like flies with the same bug, even before we were unpacked. This was the beginning of my fear that slowly built up.

Years later, after transferring to Ottawa and starting our journey with God, my fear slowly continued to consume me. There was a silent period in my life, though, when I thought it had disappeared by itself. Then, all of sudden, I started to get "ill" again. This time, it was associated with traveling anywhere. If I had to stay anywhere overnight, anxiety would crawl in bed with me. *Tired* is a weak word for how I felt. Exhausted, weak, and feeling hopeless, I was at a dead end.

But God always comes in and saves the day when we call out in desperation. Ladies Conference is my favorite event of the year, and it's held here in Ontario, right by the beautiful waters of Huyck's Bay. Jesus, friends, good food, a little bit of shopping, and the beautiful peace that nature offers—there really is nothing better.

That year was my first time attending a Ladies Conference with any sort of anxiety looming over me. As we sat down for the first service that evening, I could feel my body start to betray me. Darkness and despair held onto me as I envisioned another tortured night of feeling ill and restless sleep. Then I started to get angry—how could this happen at my favorite event? *Jesus is here*, I thought. *Why am I dealing with this?* At my point of desperation, I began to call on the name of Jesus and asked that He heal me from my anxiety and torment. As praise lifted from my mouth, I could feel His healing hands touching my mind, body, and soul. I knew that there was something different in me, that He had worked on me that night.

In our room after the service, I went right to sleep. That might not seem like a big deal, but for someone like me, that was huge. The version of me before being touched by Jesus that evening would have rolled around all night, feeling sick.

When I think of how long it took me to reach out to Jesus, I'm reminded of the man who was healed at the pool of Bethesda. The history of the pool is of utmost importance when examining this lesson. People who were sick would wait for the moving of the water, and when that happened, everyone would try to be the first to jump in. The first to touch the water would be made well. In this lesson, we learn of a certain man who had been waiting thirty-eight years to be made well. Yes, he had lived that long with his infirmity. The problem for him was that someone always beat him to the water, so he had no chance of being healed. Jesus stops to speak with him:

> When Jesus saw him lie, and knew that he had been
> now a long time in that case, he saith unto him,
> Wilt thou be made whole? (John 5:6)

28

What a question! This man didn't answer the question; he simply explained why he was unable to get into the pool. I imagine Jesus thinking, *That is not what I asked you. My question was, do you want to be well?* Perhaps that man did believe he answered the question; obviously, he did want to be well. He'd been attempting to be first in the pool for years!

Although it may seem evident to you and me, this man was not looking to Jesus for his healing. He was waiting for his chance to get into that pool. This is why I believe Jesus asked him if he wanted to be well. This man was so focused on getting into the pool for his healing that he nearly missed the revelation of who was standing right in front of him. Think about it: everyone else was sitting there, waiting for the water to move for their healing. Little did they know that Jesus, our Healer, was right beside them.

Today, when we are afflicted with something, many times we sit by the pool, waiting for our turns. During that time, Jesus is waiting for us, wondering if we really want to be well.

Do you? He told the man to rise, pick up his bed, and simply walk. A small action, but an action always is required of you in a healing. If you study healings performed by Jesus in scripture, you'll see they require an action on the person's part. When this man was healed, Jesus didn't just say to him, "You are healed." He asked him to rise, pick up his bed, and walk. This man had faith to receive the healing. What would have happened if he had replied, "I can't get up. My infirmity does not allow me to walk"? By his faith in Jesus, he rose to his feet and was forever changed.

That night at the Ladies Conference, I rose to my feet to meet Jesus, lifted up my burdens to Him, and walked with the power of God within me. I claimed the healing that He wanted to give me. The change in me was undeniable, and I will forever hold that moment close to my heart when Jesus and I shared that night. How wonderful is it that we can have a personal relationship with Him?

A healing of the mind is perpetual, which means it occurs repeatedly. Our circumstances are forever changing, and they repeatedly affect our minds. One thing that is constant is God's promise. If He has promised us a healing, then we must believe that it will be and believe it is fulfilled.

A year later, our world was turned upside down by the COVID-19 pandemic. At the beginning of the pandemic, we were expecting our fourth baby and were moving into a new, larger home to give us more room. God walked us through this challenging move in a time of great uncertainty. It was just on the cusp of everything closing down and lockdowns being put into place; about a week later, everything was locked down. We were thankful to have moved right before life became even more complicated. In a way, we were also thankful for this time we had been given to slowly unpack our new home and spend time as a family together.

We would have liked to have friends and family over, but this was a special time like no other, and I will hold it close to my heart forever. For months and months—which turned into a year—we were "forced" to stay home and spend time together. Esmée, our fourth baby, arrived that first summer, and our whole family unit was delighted to have that time together. We walked outside on trails more than we ever have, and bonfires in our backyard became a common activity. It was only a five-minute walk to a small beach, so that meant that we spent a lot of time enjoying the view and water. I felt blessed beyond measure to have been gifted that time with my little family.

After a year and a half of lockdown, restrictions finally started to lift. For me, one of the most exciting aspects was the ability to attend in-person Bible study and church again. Another big win was that we could finally gather with family and friends. Everything seemed to be smooth sailing and going just as I imagined it would.

Then, out of nowhere, I started to feel anxiety creep into my life again. This time, though, it was different—I didn't know where it was coming from. I'd be fine all day; then, as the evening rolled around, anxiety would get a tight grip on me. Even odder was that there was no event tied to it, as there had been like in the past.

Driving to Bible study the first few times, I felt the tightening in my chest, heavy breathing, and nausea. I thought, *What in the world is happening to me?* I had no idea what to think of this. I previously had experienced nausea but never the other two symptoms. One night while Jon was away at Men's Conference was perhaps the worst. I was up all night, battling the anxiety. I'd fall asleep for five minutes, then wake up, startled and having a hard time breathing—and don't forget the nausea. It was torture at its finest. I had no idea how to control this or what to do with it.

The next morning, I crawled out of bed to get up with Esmée, who was only one year old. I made coffee, turned a show on TV for her, and lay on the couch in utter defeat. This was new territory for me. I was at a complete loss. I lay there in a type of exhaustion that I'd never felt before.

Anxiety takes everything you have and then some, leaving you with nothing to draw from.

This went on for some time before I finally admitted that something needed to be done. I was beyond tired and was starting to look sick. I could not live like this anymore. The thought that I kept pushing back was, *If Jesus healed me, why am I dealing with this?* I felt like a fraud and was angry with my situation. Funny enough, I felt no anger toward Jesus; it was more toward myself. I felt like I had failed or done something wrong.

Admitting the problem is the first step to finding a solution. That's what I finally did. Once that was out of the way, I felt mentally liberated to work on a solution. Slowly I came to a realization that healing was daily. Jesus had given me all the tools I needed to win this battle. I just needed to learn how to walk in His healing daily. I began to see every day as a blessing. Every morning as the sun rose and I was breathing, there was something to be thankful for. Some mornings, I would pull myself out of bed, crawling because of the night I'd had. But I turned my suffering into joy by being grateful that a new day had begun—the sun was up, and so was I!

> From the rising of the sun unto the going down of the
> same the Lord's name is to be praised. (Psalm 113:3)

I saw that every morning was a promise from the Lord that I was going to be OK. The morning became a sacred time for me. It became my morning routine to wake up earlier than the kids and have my time with the Lord. I read my Bible, spent time in prayer, and relished the opportunity to be alone with God. Because I have seen and felt deep darkness in my life, I know how sacred is the promise that light holds. I have learned to hold on to that with every fiber of my being, clinging to what it represents for me.

My sunrise might be completely different from what it is for you, but I can promise you that you have a sunrise to get you through each day, to walk you through your daily healing. Believe that your victory is around the corner, just like that sunrise that keeps showing up. Jordan St. Cyr has a song called "Victory" that speaks about Jesus being our victory within all we do, within the storms and darkness we encounter. I could have chosen a slow song for this chapter, but I felt that "Victory" suited it best. The song is upbeat and full of life, promise, and victory, which is exactly what we need when we are going through anxiety. Get up and jump a little. Claim what the Lord has for you, with the belief that it is already done.

There is a school of thought in Christianity that because we have Jesus, we should not need any medication or counseling for mental health. I wholeheartedly disagree with that idea; in fact, I believe that God gave us doctors for a reason. Just as we see a doctor for a physical illness, we should see one for a mental illness. If we can get sick in the body, then we can get sick in the mind too.

In the fall when everything started to open up again, I finally talked with my doctor about my struggle. I hadn't planned to say anything to him, but Jon was there and spoke up. I held the shame that most of us have with mental struggles. *Maybe if I don't talk about it, the struggle will just go away.*

The doctor asked what my daily life looked like. What was my routine? At that time, I had already started to implement the tools I knew to use to win this battle. I was working out five days a week and eating healthfully. Sleep was usually pretty good, minus the nights when anxiety hit me. Self-care was a regular part of my life. Reading was one of my favorite pastimes, among others.

He looked puzzled for a minute and was not quite sure he could recommend adding or changing anything in my life. Finally, after questioning me about what an anxiety episode looked like for me, he recommended medication. I was to take it only when I was having a hard time falling asleep, and nausea struck.

A sense of relief flowed within me. I didn't feel so alone. It was comforting to know that what I was going through could be helped. Peace from God also consumed me in that moment, like He was telling me, *This is OK. You need this right now. You don't need to be ashamed to get help. You are not meant to do this alone.*

My doctor felt comfortable with prescribing medication because, according to him, I was already doing all that I could do to fight this. I believe that the Lord feels that way about this particular help as well. My true healing is in Jesus, walking daily with Him and applying all the tools He's given me, but I know that sometimes we need extra help. That's why it was put there.

Fear looks like darkness; anxiety feels like you are trapped in a dark, deep, never-ending hole. You can be a muscle-building, cross-fit, everyday lifter, but when anxiety hits, that all goes down the drain. The mind will take everything you have and pin you down to the ground with an all-consuming weakness.

Remember that fear is a liar that tells you that darkness will never lift. This is not what the Lord has promised you. Every new sunrise is His promise to be praised. Whatever your sunrise is, hold on to it with your life and know that God will lift you out of that dark place. Every morning when you place your feet on the ground, you've already won! You're up and have the opportunity to praise God for the sunrise and the breath within you. Now, walk perpetually in your promised healing.

1. "Do you want to be well?" This is what Jesus asked the man at the Bethesda pool. What healing do you need? That perhaps you've been looking for in the wrong place? Can you answer Jesus's question and ask for your healing?

2. What is your "sunrise"? How can you implement this into your daily life to walk in your healing?

3. Listen to the song "Victory" by Jordan St. Cyr. Turn it up, jump around, and claim your God-given victory! What does your victory look like? Write a short paragraph about it.

4

SUPERFOOD MIND

The *Merriam-Webster Dictionary* defines a superfood as follows:

> a food (such as salmon, broccoli, or blueberries) that is rich in compounds (such as antioxidants, fiber, or fatty acids) considered beneficial to a person's health

A superfood is any food that is full of the nutrients needed to maintain good health. It may be a food that can offer various health benefits at the same time.

I'm not a person who only buys superfoods or takes the time to look for them. It's true, however, that we are what we eat. The food we eat has a direct effect on our minds and how well they function. For example, a person who is living with untreated celiac disease often will complain about brain fog. That isn't the only symptom or the worst, but it is present nonetheless.

It blows my mind that people can experience brain fog because they eat gluten! Children who are diagnosed with ADHD or ADD are often told to cut back on certain foods to help with learning. Parents of autistic children may try to eliminate certain foods from the children's diets, as that has proven beneficial for their behavior, which is controlled by the mind.

I hope to help you learn how to feed your mind. Remember that controlling your mind is foundational, but what you feed it is just as important. If you don't nourish the mind, you can't properly control it. What you feed your mind will affect your words or actions in a positive or negative way.

I didn't always have healthy eating habits, but I implemented healthy eating in my life about five years ago. My motivation to do this was triggered by my mental state and a busy lifestyle. I was a mom of three, working a nine-to-five job, five days a week, while trying to maintain my mental health. I hadn't given much thought to what I was eating and the effect it could have on me. I'm going to apologize now for the next statement, as I know many people struggle with their weight—I have been genetically blessed with a slim figure that allows me to eat what I want. My dad is tall and lanky, so I came by this honestly. I also have a sweet tooth—give me a bucket of cotton candy, and I'll be pleased. Breakfast for dinner is a favorite go-to because it usually includes pancakes or waffles with all the fixings.

It was only when I tried to juggle full-time work and mommy-ing that I looked into the theory of healthy eating. If I'm going to do something, usually I do a ton of research on it. There needs to be purpose behind my actions. Following my careful research, I could see that what we eat affects our mental states. Sugar was my biggest battle; my diet was full of all things sweet.

When the body is used to consuming sugar, it becomes addicted to it, and it then requires a constant supply of it to function. It's no different from caffeine in the morning that gives you a boost of energy to get going. Sugar plays with our moods, hormone levels, stress levels, and memories, to name a few. Something so seemingly harmless can affect us at a very deep level.

As I started to eliminate my "kryptonite" from my diet, some days were difficult, as my body craved sugar. As time went on, however, things started to level out—and my skin started to clear up too. I previously had regular breakouts, but now, those were few and far between. My energy levels stabilized, and I seemed to have more of it, which was groundbreaking; previously, sugar had given me my oomph. Most noteworthy, however, is that my mind felt healthier. Things were clearer, and I had fewer mood crashes and less depression or anxiety.

Sugar is not the only food that affects the mind; gluten is another big-ticket item. Try to figure out which food triggers your mind to spiral. A healthy diet filled with vegetables, fruit, protein, grains, and healthy fats is a good place to start. Don't overcomplicate the process. (It can seem more daunting than it actually is.) Try eliminating or scaling back on sugar or caffeine, and see the difference that makes in your life. Drink water, water, and more water. Hydration is important to a healthy, functioning mind; that's not just for athletes. As my grandmother would say, use the KISS principle, which means to keep it super simple. No need to go to the health food store and buy all the gluten-free and sugar-free items. Don't starve yourself because you've overcomplicated your diet in your mind and have no idea where to start. Just start with *something*; that is what counts.

I suggest doubling your current water intake, scale back on sugar or unhealthy carbs, and fill your diet with vegetables and fruits. If you don't have time to cut up fresh vegetables every evening, use frozen—nothing wrong with that! Are you rushed in the morning with no time to make a healthy breakfast? Make yourself overnight oats in the fridge. Grab a mason jar, add your oats with whichever dairy you prefer, then add the extras. Whether that is maple syrup, fruit, nuts, or chocolate chips. The internet has an abundance of variations for overnight oats. You might think, *I already know all of this. These are no-brainer tips.* My question to you is this: are you applying them to your daily life? It is one thing to know something and another thing to actually live it. I'm not a certified nutritionist, but you don't need to hear all the science behind which fruit contains which vitamins. You only need to start on your road to building your superfood mind. I've simplified it in a way that is understandable to anyone looking to commence his or her journey to healing.

In our home, we have this thing we call *time*—it's the amount of game time our kids are allotted every week. Usually, it stays the same from week to week, but sometimes, it can go either up or down. During a normal school week, our children are not allowed to play their video games or watch television. This may seem harsh, but in this era where electronics are everywhere, I feel this restriction is necessary for my children's well-being. They use computers at school more and more, and everything else is connected in some shape or form to electronics. *Time* can be taken away as a consequence, or we will allow them more time if it's a special weekend or as a reward. My kids consistently tell me how unfair this is and that their friends get to play anytime they want.

Have you ever seen kids who have just come off their video games or just finished watching television all day? They act like zombies—creatures who are slowly emerging from another world. Look into their eyes, and you'll notice they're glazed over, and the kids' moods have changed—but not a good change in mood; they are grumpy. They just got to do what they wanted to do so badly, and now they are in a bad mood. Go figure.

When my mom didn't want me watching too much television, she would say, "You don't want your brain turning to mush." That saying was widely used back then, and I still say it to my children. I'm guilty of watching too much television or scrolling on social media for far longer than I should have. My husband and I have binged-watched a television series on a Friday night, for example, only to look at the time and realize how late it is. Funny thing is that when we do that, I'm not tired at midnight. My body is sore, and I feel mentally exhausted, but I'm not tired enough to fall asleep. We haven't done that in such a long time, as I really do hate feeling like mush.

Have you scrolled too long on social media? I think it's interesting that we call it *scrolling*, as that is exactly what it is. We are not truly reading or taking in the information. Our eyes are simply following the screen, but our minds are not working as they should. We are not feeding our minds; we're losing our "muscle mass." When we become ill and stay in bed for a day or longer, our muscle mass begins decreasing. The same idea can apply to our minds when we don't use them or "feed" them correctly. Our minds lose muscle mass as we choose not to exercise them daily with the proper tools.

If you have never practiced exercising and feeding the mind, then you may not be aware of what you are missing. Similarly, a person who has never worked out has no idea how great that change will make him or her feel. Trust me—as you feed your mind, you will slowly become addicted to the way it makes you feel. You also will notice the difference if you divert from a well-fed and exercised mind. The question is, how do we feed and exercise the mind?

The Word of God is one piece of equipment we have to exercise our minds. Through reading and studying the Word, we learn who God is and what He wants for us. The Bible you hold in your hand is man-written but wholly inspired by God. The content of it is not instruction only for those in the biblical era; it is still applicable today and should be put into practice.

The apostles had the extreme privilege of following Jesus and, thus, spoke to and learned from Him directly. When I think about meeting Jesus, I become speechless and am awed by the very thought of it. I read the Word, and it speaks to me. I have questions, and I often am blown away by the power it contains.

> For the word of God is alive and active. Sharper than any double-edged sword, it penetrates even to dividing soul and spirit, joints and marrow; it judges the thoughts and attitudes of the heart. (Hebrews 4:12)

Looking at that scripture confirms how alive the Word of God is in our lives. This verse also says that it is active—wow! If the Word of God is active, then we need to actively read it and apply it to our lives. We need to use it to fight our battles, as it is sharper than any double-edged sword and is the best way to confront adversity in our lives.

God's Word is our daily bread for our spiritual hunger. It nurtures our minds, bodies, and souls.

> But he answered and said, It is written, Man shall not live by bread alone, but by every word that proceedeth out of the mouth of God. (Matthew 4:4)

Jesus tells us in Matthew 4:4 that we cannot live only by the food we eat; we need the Word of God. The food we consume is a temporal fix to our hunger, but His Word fulfills an eternal hunger daily.

There is a reason that God gave us the written Word. It's not only that He knew we would need it but that it would be a lighthouse in our lives. A lighthouse has two main purposes: it is used as a navigational aid and as a warning to boats of surrounding dangerous waters. As we walk daily, our minds need a constant navigational aid; we are not able to do this on our own. We might believe we can at times, but that often results in our becoming lost in the darkness. Our minds require guidance on the content we are to focus on. If we don't take that step, then our minds inevitably will wander.

The word *wander* can be described as aimlessly walking into unknown or known territory. I've told my children, "Please don't wander off," because I don't want them to get lost. We all wander off the path at times in our lives, and with that, we face danger. One response to danger is to eliminate it or fight against it with whatever weapon we may have. Hebrews 4:12 tells us that the Word of God is sharper than any double-edged sword. We should have it stored away and ready for action. Read the Word daily, hide it in your heart and mind, and meditate on it as you go about your day. Write scripture on sticky notes and place them around your house—whatever you have to do to have access to it at all times. You have to start somewhere.

The Word is for everyone; it was meant to be read. The first time reading the Bible can be intimidating. I remember my first attempt at it. I've heard that each time you read the entire Bible, you learn something new, and I've found that is the gospel truth! As years went on, I read and studied the Bible more. It suddenly became less about checking off a box and more about God revealing Himself to me through His Word. I love to think of the Word as God's tangible heartbeat. Through it, we can feel and connect with His deepest desires, His likes and dislikes, and His purpose for us and His kingdom. Similar to God's being able to discern what is in our hearts and minds, we have a very real way to do the same with Him.

As the Word is a form of gateway to God's heart, desires, and plans, prayer is our opportunity to communicate with a very accessible God. I'd like to suggest that prayer is a conversation, and what is the basis of a good conversation? It's when two people are talking, not just one. If you are doing all the talking in what you believe to be a conversation, then I'm sorry, but you are simply talking at that person. He or she is listening, but you don't allow that person to respond. A stereotypical example is when a wife speaks with her husband. There are times when she talks his ear off without realizing he hasn't said anything yet. Many husbands are happy to listen and not say much, but this is not so with God. In prayer, you should speak to Him and then wait for His response. It may take some time, and you will have to be still and listen closely, but God wants you to give Him the opportunity to speak with you.

I've been in conversations in which the other person does not stop talking at all. I just sit there, nodding my head and smiling. Every so often I try to get a word in, but as the French would say, *c'est impossible!* Or I might be "allowed" to begin a sentence but not finish it because that person unknowingly cuts me off. Have you ever come to God in this way? We just have so much to say to Him and perhaps so many requests. All the while, God just sits there, chin placed in His hand (at least, that's how I picture Him), waiting for us to be quiet.

Maybe you stop talking for a minute, as God gears up to speak, then you storm back in, saying, "And another thing!" We need to allow God the chance to speak into our lives and situations. That requires us to be still and simply enter into His presence.

Prayer and the Word of God work together; they go hand in hand. Through the Word, we are able to discern what God may be trying to tell us. We've already established that many thoughts and feelings go through our minds each day. If we have no knowledge of God's Word, it is very difficult for us to tell which thoughts or feelings are of God and which are not. Not every feeling we get is from God, which makes it extremely important to be able to recognize God's voice in our lives. The enemy is a liar that tries to speak things into our lives and minds. Without the Word of God, we may not be able to see the lies.

A superfood mind will use prayer daily to seek strength and wisdom and to have the ability to fight against what may come against it. Prayer with God is free access to our own therapist twenty-four hours a day. Pouring out our hearts to God is therapeutic, as is knowing we can fully come to Him and that He is there with arms wide open. In my personal experience with anxiety, I have found that when my mind is anxious, I close up. I stop talking, my jaw becomes stiff, and I forget to pray.

We can become anxious and panic in the moment; it's as if we don't know how to respond, so we are somewhat paralyzed. Through the ritual of daily prayer and speaking the Word of God in our lives, we feed the mind with the food it requires to stay strong in times of trials. We have instant access to God at all times. Wi-Fi connections these days usually are very fast, but that doesn't compare to the access you have to God. All you need to do is speak His name once, and you instantly have his attention. In fact, He already knew you were coming to speak with Him.

As described in the New Testament, Jesus went into prayer often. He would slip away early in the morning.

42

> And in the morning, rising up a great while before
> day, he went out, and departed into a solitary place,
> and there he prayed. (Mark 1:35)

Before Jesus started the day, He prayed alone. It was still dark, and everyone was asleep. That was the point, though—He could go and be alone with God. You can find a special connection when you go to prayer early in the morning. Perhaps that's because it really feels as if it's just you and God. You can find strength for the day through this type of prayer. If Jesus found it a necessary and vital action, then how much more do we need to build prayer into our daily lives? So much that it becomes a habit that we do without thinking.

Prayer is not for when you have a need. God will meet your needs, and it is important to pray for them, but this is a sliver of what prayer should look like. If you were to converse with someone who only asks you for favors all the time, wouldn't you grow tired of that conversation?

In a solid relationship, we lift each other up, share our deepest sorrows and successes, thank each other, and, at times, simply listen to each other. Our relationships with God should look the same; we should be praying and converse about all things.

When I'm on a walk, I often enter into continual praise. While doing the dishes, I often pour my heart out to God. I talk to Him like I would talk to a friend, and this allows me to open up in the simplest way.

You don't need to be eloquent, or to have a PhD in prayer, or to write it out and then rehearse it before speaking to Him. You just need to come to Him and trust Him with all your mind, soul, and heart. "Lord, I need You today" is enough. "Lord, You know my heart and struggles. Please help me"—sometimes this is all you need to say. Begin today with the simplest prayer, and watch your mind flourish as He works within you.

Feeding your mind should be a consistent action, which means you don't start your day with prayer and then forget about it for the rest of the day—this is often a common mistake when building the mind. *Started my day in prayer—check! Read the Word—check! Healthy breakfast—check!* It's only 9:00 a.m., and you've already checked off your list. Then you just go about the rest of your day without a thought to your mind. You might say, "I don't understand. I started the day right." That's perfect and good for you, but you need to be intentional about the rest of your day too. Instead of scrolling on social media, maybe you could listen to a podcast that nourishes your mind and gets you thinking.

What about the books you read? I enjoy a good mindless read from time to time, but when I read something that really nurtures and works my mind, it is empowering. How do you end your day? Hands up if you just turn on a show and zone out. Absolutely nothing wrong with that, but I have found that finishing the day with a devotion sets the tone for the night. Your devotion doesn't need to be an hour long; ten to fifteen minutes is enough. This will allow you to wind down and focus on God one more time before finishing the day that He has so graciously carried you through. Just as the sunrise brings a new day of mercies, the sunset proves His grace toward you in another day that is completed. Starting and ending your day with God allows you to continually walk in the Spirit.

> This I say then, Walk in the Spirit, and ye shall not fulfil the lust of the flesh. For the flesh lusteth against the Spirit, and the Spirit against the flesh: and these are contrary the one to the other: so that ye cannot do the things that ye would. But if ye be led of the Spirit, ye are not under the law. (Galatians 5:16–18)

When we allow ourselves to walk in the Spirit, we can walk in our daily healing, believing and knowing from whom it comes. The flesh tells us otherwise, but the Spirit will guide us to the promises that God has for us. The flesh tells us that we don't need any of that and will often direct us on the wrong path, walking us away from our healing. By beginning and finishing every day with God, however, we will have the strength to feed our minds that "superfood" it very much needs.

The song I chose for this chapter is called "Look What You've Done" by Tasha Layton. The title almost speaks for itself—it's about what God has done in our lives. I love to sing with all my might, declaring what He has done for me and will continue to do.

As you feed your mind, and you see the change in yourself, you are allowed to celebrate that with Him. I invite you to claim that today, and as you progress, have your little dance party with the Lord, praising Him for all He's done. Don't forget to praise Him for what He will do—He's not done with any of us yet!

1. Think about your daily diet. Are you consuming too much or too little of certain foods, which could be affecting your mind? If so, write out your game plan below. Remember not to overcomplicate it. Just start!

2. What does a regular day look like for you? How can you implement the Word in your daily life? Write down a time that you are able to commit to reading the Word.

3. Start a prayer list. It can feel daunting when you don't know where to start, but this will help you enter into focused prayer. Write down all the things you want to praise God for too.

4. Listen to "Look What You've Done" by Tasha Layton. Write down all the healings you are claiming, and sing this song, praising God in advance.

5

WHOSE YOKE?

As I've mentioned, in the middle of the pandemic, we welcomed our fourth child, and our house got busier than ever. It was a good busy, though. Our three other children were fourteen, eleven, and nine at the time. That kind of age difference offers a different dynamic than when they were all toddlers. Our three oldest begged us to get a dog a few months after Esmée was born. At first, my answer was a hard no, as this didn't sound like a great idea with a new baby. We all knew who would end up taking care of an animal in the home; parents get stuck with the tasks the kids don't do.

My kids were persistent, though, and asked that it be their Christmas gift. The begging started to wear me down, especially since I have a soft spot for dogs. I could relate to my children wanting a dog; every kid should experience the love in owning a dog.

You've probably guessed that we got a dog. Jon drove five and a half hours with our oldest, Liam, to pick up the puppy. Liam had no idea where they were going. Jon didn't tell Liam the big news until they arrived. The same day, they made the trip back home, making it a eleven-hour drive in one day.

During the pandemic, apparently it was a popular idea to get a dog, so it wasn't easy to find one near us. Our other two kids,

Novalee and Cohen, were elated when Liam walked in with a beautiful golden retriever puppy. We named him Moby, and he was absolutely perfect—everything that I thought a golden would look like. I chose that breed because I'd heard how great goldens are with families. They have a kind and loving demeanor.

You might think I was brave (or nuts) for getting a puppy with a five-month-old baby at home, but I knew that I'd be home to train the puppy properly; I had the time to devote to such an undertaking. Moby was adorable, and the kids had a great time playing with him, minus the ankle biting and jumping as he grew older. Then Moby developed a behavior that caught us completely off guard. Every time we fed him, he got defensive and aggressive if someone approached him or his food. Eventually, he went from growling to raising his lips in aggression and then almost biting one of us.

As time went on, he'd exhibit this behavior when he had a bone that he loved or any item he valued. I'd hoped it was just a phase, but it seemed to be getting worse, and with no experience with this, I didn't know what to do. Completely baffled and heartbroken—I thought we'd have to give him away—we tried one last thing; we hired a dog trainer and behavior specialist.

I am so thankful that we made that decision. Our dog trainer was incredible and very knowledgeable about why Moby behaved as he did. Golden retrievers are extremely sensitive beings, and we figured out that Moby was a very sensitive dog. (Jon was less than impressed when he learned that we had a "sensitive" dog. He'd wanted a "man's dog," and now he was stuck with a dog that was overly sensitive.)

The trainer taught us about "trigger stacking," which is an innate reaction that dogs have to their environment; some experience this more than others. In a nutshell, trigger stacking is when the dog is faced with situations that excite or stress him, one after another, causing him to enter a "red zone." For example, a new visitor comes into the home; then the kids start running around; somebody throws a ball; a toddler pulls the dog's tail; other children are playing with toys; then perhaps the dog is cornered. The triggers continue to stack up until he can no longer take it. In this red zone, he doesn't think before reacting, and that is usually when the dog can lose it.

Basically, it's a mental overload for the dog. It's important to be alert and aware of this behavior and know when the situations around him are too much to handle. As his stress amps up, he gives off signs through his face and body language that we must tune into. For example, when a dog is stressed, he gets a look like he's smiling—creases form around his jawline and his mouth is a tad open.

The important element of trigger stacking is that the "blow up" is completely preventable. If we had realized that Moby was getting stressed, we could have provided the solution, which would be to remove him from the situation and place him in a safe space to recharge alone.

Are you wondering why I'm talking about the behavior of a dog? Well, trigger stacking does not just apply to dogs. I am suggesting that every normal human is prone to trigger stacking in his or her daily life. Try to imagine this situation with me: You wake up startled, realizing you've missed the alarm, which also means you have no time to yourself this morning to pray or read the Word. Why did you miss the alarm? You were completely exhausted from the day you had yesterday, and today, there is even more on your plate. As you head downstairs to open the cupboard to make your coffee, you suddenly remember that you used the last of the coffee yesterday. You think, *That's OK. I'll make myself a cup of tea.*

As the water boils, you begin to put lunches together for the day. The hissing from the kettle stops you. As you pour, hot water splashes out of the cup and all over the counter. Thankful that you didn't get burned, you keep moving. Ah, that first sip is perfection, exactly what you needed. Just then, one of the kids stampedes downstairs, yelling, "Mommy, Mommy!"

Back to reality, you keep making the lunches and prep breakfast in unison. You can hear the two other kids upstairs, yelling about not being able to find socks, and you snicker a bit because you told them last night to fold their clothes. The kids are zooming all around you, packing their lunches while you think about your big to-do list for the day.

Ping! Your phone goes off, and as you pick it up, one of the kids asks you a question that can't wait. Your try to read the message and answer your child at the same time. Your mind is already in a haze, and it's only 7:15 a.m.

"Hurry up—go brush your teeth and comb your hair!" you yell as you try to take another sip of your tea, secretly wishing it was the coffee you were anticipating since opening your eyes this morning. Finally, everyone's bag is packed, teeth are brushed, shoes are on, and they have eaten their breakfast.

As you usher them outside to wait for the bus, you give them a big hug, telling them, "I love you." You breathe in deeply as you think about your next step for this busy day. Just then, your toddler pulls on your leg, asking for a snack. Your to-do list is long, and you wonder how you will complete it by the end of the day. But you must; this is what you do. Your worth is found in how much you accomplish.

OK, then you decide, *I'll start with cleaning the bathrooms and floors. After that, I have to tackle some of the work I've been meaning to do. Oh no, what about my workout?* You tell yourself that's OK; maybe you will have time for that tomorrow.

Starting with the bathrooms and floors, you just keep moving, and before you know it, you need to make lunch for your toddler. It would be much easier if you didn't have to make lunch, and you could keep on with the list. As the day wears on, you keep pushing yourself. You are mentally and physically exhausted, and the kids aren't even home from school yet. The day ends; you flop your tired and worn-out body into your bed with little energy for your devotion. You think, *At least I got my list done today. That is something to be proud of. Maybe I can find time for myself tomorrow.* When you don't find time yourself, the accumulation of the responsibilities, results in a form of trigger stacking.

Are you employed outside the home? Perhaps your schedule is forever changing because of shift work. Maybe your job is to serve and protect, to walk out into the darkness as everyone sleeps comfortably in their homes. Kiss your partner and tuck your kids into bed as their day ends, but yours is just about to begin. As you step out into the night, you wonder what trials you may face. Your mind cannot unsee what you've seen.

Your erratic lifestyle does not allow you to create a balance or routine. You wear a bulletproof vest, carry a gun, and keep your hand on your baton, but that still does not protect your mind from the events you've seen. Answering a 911 call, you never know if the person actually wants you there. You never want to end things in physical combat, but at the end of the day, you just want to make it home.

Your partner asked you to stay safe, and with every fiber of your being, you try to make that a reality. This is not just a job but a calling; that is why you continue to show up for work every day. You walk into the office, prepared to catch up on last night's paperwork, only to get called out right away.

And so, the night continues in this rhythm, one call after another, and you know that no paperwork will get done tonight. But whether or not you have time tonight, it will have to get done. Not only do you have to live through these disasters, but you also have to relive them by putting together a detailed file.

You walk into a home to find a toddler sitting on the floor by herself, crying, filthy, and in desperate need of a diaper change. The parents are passed out at the kitchen table, too intoxicated to notice that you just walked in. This is the third time that you've come back to this home, and you take the child, who will be placed with a foster family. Anger wells up inside as you attempt to understand how a parent could let this happen, and you wish that there was more you could do.

Next, you attend to a car crash, where several people have lost their lives and are unrecognizable from the injuries; they don't even look human anymore. That image will haunt you forever. You know that falling asleep, come morning, will not be easy after seeing this wreck. A few more calls, and your shift comes to an end. You'd like nothing better than to forget what you've witnessed tonight.

You need to wake up earlier, as your child has a recital at school the next day that she's begged you to attend. Your "night" will be short. You know the kind of day your partner will have, trying to keep the kids quiet so you can sleep. You try to shut off your mind and clear the images, but you have no idea how a person is supposed to deal with this. It feels like your mind is never at rest, and you are constantly in combat mode. *How do I shut it off?* you wonder. This is what you signed up for, but when do you get to rest?

The pictures I painted are only a glimpse of what any one person could be going through daily. Perhaps you are not a stay-at-home mom or even a parent. That doesn't change the message. You may be working full time from home, surrounded by your work daily as you "live" in the office. Your reality may be that you travel a long distance each day to get to work, only to arrive home exhausted. Perhaps you are a caregiver, taking care of your parents or any other loved one, and your life is consumed with giving yourself to others.

Whatever our particular realities, there is no doubt that we are all racing to the next task on our list. Society has built us in such a way that we feel that is what we are expected to do. Our sense of self and worth is found in what we do, instead of who we are and belong to. We accumulate the weight of every single day, essentially trigger stacking within our routines.

Do you allow yourself to keep going, even though you can sense the signs that are asking for rest? Whatever your walk in life, if you replaced some words in either story, that is likely how you feel at the end of the day.

We all have a purpose, and we all have obligations that need to be fulfilled. But the question is, how can we live in a state of perpetual rest while going through the motions of day-to-day life?

The Bible story of Martha and Mary offers perfect symbolism

for this particular concept. As Jesus and His disciples were traveling to a village, Martha invited them into her home. Scripture states that Martha was extremely preoccupied with everything she had to do, so much so that Martha complained to Jesus about Mary not helping her with the tasks that had to be completed.

Mary was awestruck with wonder about what Jesus had to say. She basked in His presence and was caught up in this encounter she was experiencing. Following Martha's plea for help:

> And Jesus answered and said unto her, Martha, Martha, thou art careful and troubled about many things:
>
> But one thing is needful: and Mary hath chosen that good part, which shall not be taken away from her. (Luke 10:41–42)

Martha had chosen to get caught up with the day-to-day things that she thought needed to be finished, while Mary made the decision to rest in Jesus's presence and listen to what He had to say. Unbeknownst to Martha, she may have been trigger stacking that day, when she should have spent time focusing on Jesus.

Can you think of a season or time that you've been a Martha? We all have, at one time or another. We're so busy attempting to finish or start what we believe needs to be done that we forget that what He really wants—for us to take the time to stop and rest in Him. Perhaps we're trying to prove to Him that we are worthy by doing all the things, but all He really wants is that relationship with us. If we can find the time to rest in Jesus, then He will give us the time to champion through. If we can put Him before any task, He will also show us what is truly important.

Maybe you are busy trying to fill the void that should be occupied by Him completely. The busier you are, the less time you have to think about how you feel empty and exhausted every day.

By doing this, you are telling him that He's not enough, although you most likely don't do it purposely. Nonetheless, your overfilled days declare that the honor to be in His presence is not enough. This may seem harsh; maybe you think, *That's not what I'm trying to tell Him at all.*

We do it subconsciously, then apologize for not fitting time in to be in His presence daily. If He were enough, we would prioritize our time to rest in Him, knowing that our strength comes from Him.

Martha did not believe that her actions were wrong; in fact, she thought that Mary was wrong. The feeling of weariness on my heart and mind always seems to follow days on which I did not put God first and seek the rest only He can give me.

Martha needed to get her mind and heart together and achieve a state of perpetual rest. Her mind was so preoccupied that her heart was hijacked that day. Mary, on the other hand, thought with her heart and allowed her emotions to decide her actions. The heart and the mind are connected in a deeply profound way. They should work together to guide us through life.

Did you know that the vagus nerve is the longest nerve in the body? It connects from the mind to the heart, lungs, and gut. (We will focus on the connection between the mind and the heart.) The vagus nerve is a key component of the parasympathetic system, our rest-and-digest nervous system. This nerve affects our breathing, digestive systems, and heart rates. These three components affect our mental health.

Activating our vagus nerves increases *vagal tone*, which then puts our parasympathetic systems into action. We can activate the vagus nerve in several ways. We should strive for a high vagal tone, as that helps the body relax in times of stress. Some suggested techniques to increase vagal tone are singing or humming, slow deep breathing, exercising, socializing, taking probiotics, and exposing ourselves to cold.

Have you ever felt unwell and used an ice-cold facecloth to help with your unease? There is a reason it is so effective; research suggests that exposure to cold, whether through splashing cold water on your face or taking a cold shower activates, the vagus nerve. The research is ongoing as to how the vagus nerve affects mental health, but one thing is certain: the vagus nerve does affect response to stressful situations.

Remember that every action, word, or decision is run through the mind before being executed. With regard to the vagus nerve, the mind and heart are connected and affect each other. They can function either in unison or off beat. A heart and mind that speak to each other will benefit your mental, physical, and emotional state. When you are heartbroken by a circumstance in life, your mind suffers and is not capable of functioning at full capacity. Think of the common phrase "my heart is full"; a gleaming face and mind accompany that emotion.

The Lord has taught me how to be at rest in Him and in my circumstances. Through much prayer and discipline of the mind and heart, I have seen and tasted what is truly important in life. To be truly at rest in the Lord, you need to take two steps in your life. The first step is knowing whose yoke you are attempting to carry. A yoke is the wooden crosspiece that sits on the necks of two animals so that they can pull a cart together. Matthew 11:28–30 refers to the yoke that we are meant to carry:

> Come to Me, all you who labor and are heavy laden,
> and I will give you rest. Take My yoke upon you and
> learn from Me, for I am gentle and lowly in heart,
> and you will find rest for your souls. For My yoke
> is easy and My burden is light.

The yoke is meant to lighten the load for the animals that pull the cart by working together instead of alone. In this scripture, God tells us that we are to take *His* yoke because it is easy and light. How often have we forgotten whose yoke we are to carry while trying to handle the burdens that life throws at us? Not only burdens, but simply day-to-day life that slowly wears us down when we run the race alone. It also blows me away that contrary to the load we should have to carry, when we take God's yoke, the load is exponentially lighter.

Our second step to a heart and mind at rest is to know that the Lord is enough. This concept didn't cross my mind too often in my walk with God. I was satisfied in knowing that I love God and need Him, but I never reflected on the idea of His being enough. Living from a heart and mind at rest opened my eyes to the truth that we find in Him. When we live from that place long enough, we will do anything to preserve the sacredness of this relationship, even if that means we need to settle things in our hearts or eliminate certain areas of our lives. To know that He is enough is to be fully content and accept where we are and what we have in life. It is believing that nothing else matters because He sustains us *every single minute.*

These two steps will stop us from trigger stacking and creating a life of chaos in our minds. Learning that our hearts and minds are connected in a profound way will foster an attitude of intentionality. A heart that is at rest produces a mind capable of rest.

You will put first whatever your heart and soul treasure, therefore putting your mind to work in that area. Whatever you cherish in your heart will flow to your mind, activating a lifesaving cognitive response in every situation.

The song "Jireh" by Elevation Worship and Maverick City Music speaks to God's being enough in every circumstance, as we know we are loved by Him. Perhaps my favorite lines in this song are:

> So there's nothing I can do to let you down.
> It doesn't take a trophy to make you proud.

This teaches us that it is not about how much you do; it's more about the quality and state in which it's completed. God wants you to be fulfilled in Him completely because you are more than enough for Him. You can rest in knowing that without having done anything in this life, you were and are more than enough. Resting your mind is a daily task that requires you to find your worth perfectly in Him. It allows you to prevail through your day because He is carrying the load with you. His will be done in your daily life if you allow Him to intercede.

I pray that this chapter has conveyed the importance of a rested mind, not only for your everyday mental health but for your spiritual walk with God. This daily healing is not about your everyday life; it is so much bigger than that. This is about the eternal promise that you've been given!

1. Take a minute to look at your everyday life. Can you see where you might be trigger stacking? What do you plan to implement in your routine to help ease stressful moments?

2. Search your heart. Where do your mind and heart not meet up enough? Give it to God today, and pray that He will intervene in these areas.

3. What do you need to give to God or to lie down for a while to foster a mind and heart at rest?

4. Listen to "Jireh" by Elevation Worship and Maverick City Music, and bask in the Lord's presence, allowing your heart and mind to be fully content with where you are.

PART II
BODY

*The body is the vessel used to walk
toward our God-given purpose.*

6

FEARFULLY AND WONDERFULLY MADE

When a patient receives a heart transplant, that patient has a new, functioning, healthy heart, but certain lifestyle habits should be incorporated to keep the heart healthy. That same concept should be applied to the care of your body. While you may have received a healing, you need to ensure proper care of this new and improved you. In this chapter, we will look at how to feed our bodies for best performance.

"You are what you eat"—this carries a deep and profound meaning in this chapter. I pray that you will see that the previous chapters tie in with this one and the following ones after that. I hope I'll be able to convey that the mind, body, and soul are interrelated and function together to perform at the highest level that God created us to be.

Have you ever met someone and felt that a friendship with that person would last forever? From the day you met that person, you know this friendship was God-ordained. For me, that is my friendship with my dearest bestie, Shaila, also known as "my bean" or "ol' bean." Shaila and I met when I was in deep need of a friend. In the middle of our first posting, as Jon was right out of training from the Police Academy. Far from our family, we both felt like ducks out of water. I was alone, pregnant, and moving without help from friends or family when she showed up at our doorstep, ready to help us clean and unpack. She was a sure answer to my prayers; I had longed for an answer for months. Shaila is a ball of fire, energetically loving, and beyond kind. She is the true picture of how a Christian should act, as she constantly emulates the love of God toward everyone she meets. Fierce and strong, there is not much that can bring her down because of who she follows daily.

Shaila was diagnosed with rheumatoid arthritis a couple years after we met. She struggled with intense pain all over her body, sometimes every day for days on end. I felt so helpless that I only could offer her my prayers over the phone. We did not live close to each other when Shaila was diagnosed, so popping over to help in person was not possible. Her determination to not allow this disease to control her everyday life was unmatchable, even if that meant crawling out of bed every morning to go to work.

Although I couldn't be there in person, I was an ear that listened and a shoulder to lean on, especially on the most difficult days. Most important, though, was my ability to walk with her in faith, claiming and believing that God would heal her one day. In some of our conversations, we would praise God for the good days and the fact that she was still able to function, if with a limp—the pain in her body constantly changed, and on some days, walking was difficult. We praised God for her having the gift of breath and knew that her healing was coming, maybe not today but someday.

I'm reminded of the story in Luke 5:17–26, in which Jesus heals a paralyzed man. The man's friends were unable to break through the crowd surrounding Jesus; there were so many people, and they were carrying him on a mat, which must have been extremely difficult. Did they give up? No, they didn't. With all the more drive and determination, they decided to climb to a rooftop and lower the man down to Jesus, as they believed that Jesus would heal their friend. Surely the faith of the man's friends got Jesus's attention—that they were so confident of the healing that they removed what we today would call shingles from the roof.

We need friends who are willing to go to bat for us in the spiritual, no doubt more than in the physical. It's when we enter spiritual warfare for our friends and family that we see the greatest miracles! Friends and family who are not willing to accept us living with whatever ailment that consumes our minds, bodies, or souls.

Shaila was surrounded by prayers from her family and friends, who told her all the time that healing was near. If you asked her, she would confirm that she felt all the prayers that were sent up each day, lifting her up.

Shaila and her family moved to Ottawa, which, by the way, was an answer to prayer too. We had both longed to live in the same city as each other, and our dream finally came true. Not long after their arrival to the capital city of Canada, Shaila was healed from her rheumatoid arthritis.

It is extremely important that I share the way in which God healed her from this lifelong pain. God heals us in different ways, and one way is not more valid than the other. In fact, if you expect your blessing to look the same as others, you might miss out on your blessing or healing. That's because when you're solely focused on the way you think that God will bless or heal, you can fail to see that He's already answered. You've cornered yourself into a mindset that closes all other doors and possibilities.

Picture a couple who has been trying to save for a home. They've been praying for a miracle. Perhaps they've envisioned that God will bless them with the entire down payment. They're not entirely sure how that will happen, but they've decided He will provide their need in one lump sum. Because of that idea, they completely missed the blessing a few months back when their employer gave them a raise that increased their salary by a substantial amount, enough to comfortably save for their down payment and have it by the end of the year. Instead of saving the money, they lived within their new means and failed to save for their down payment. They completely missed the answer that God had provided.

Shaila started to see a naturopath/nutritionist who worked with her to change her eating habits. Many of the foods we eat cause inflammation in our bodies, but it's a hundred times worse for those afflicted with rheumatoid arthritis. This was no easy lifestyle change for Shaila to attempt, especially on her own. There were times when I thought it was too brutal. *Nobody should have to limit their eating like this*, I thought. She was to eliminate the following: processed foods, peanut butter and peanuts, caffeine, sugar, almost all dairy, and gluten. I wondered what was left to eat. Well, I was surprised; it was a lot of work and planning, but she did it—and her pain ceased! That's right; she was healed by adjusting her diet in a way that eliminated all inflammation in her body.

God touched her and healed in a way that was unexpected, but it was very clear to her that this was her healing. This is the perfect testament to God requiring us to do our part, and He'll do the rest. That type of diet isn't for everyone, but it's important to realize that food directly affects our health. There is not an ounce of doubt in me or Shaila that God healed and did a miracle in her body. He just had her change to clean eating habits because her previous diet was causing harm. Through that lifestyle change, Shaila was able to claim the full healing that God had waiting for her.

How is she doing today? The healing she received is still present! In fact, she would testify that, based on recent blood tests, no inflammation was detected whatsoever.

Remember that the food we feed our bodies affects our everyday lives, perhaps more than we can imagine. Food can act as fuel, or it weigh us down, making it difficult to accomplish everyday tasks. Because we eat every day, we have the opportunity to fuel our bodies with healthy food.

Ever since I can remember, my grandfather has started his day with a bowl of oatmeal. I have fond memories of him enjoying a bowl of piping-hot oatmeal when I visited the farm as a young child. Do you know why he chose to eat oatmeal every morning? Because he was very aware of the day ahead and knew that his body required a breakfast full of substance and nutrition. He also knew that as a person ages, he should pay a little more attention to his health.

When I would visit, he always surprised my sister and me with Froot Loops and other sugary cereals. We would beam from ear to ear and were overjoyed, as my mother didn't buy that for us. Sweets have always been like kryptonite for me. When I feel low or sad, I nibble on a chocolate bar. Low energy? I chow down on a sweet snack to get my blood sugar levels back up. When I became old enough to make my own dietary decisions, I considered sugar as a food group. I was giving myself a temporary pick-me-up, because we all know about the sugar crash that comes after the high.

About five years ago, I started to change my eating habits to improve my physical, emotional, and mental health. I was trying to maintain a very busy lifestyle—working full time in the core of Ottawa and balancing a home life with three children. I realized that if I was going to succeed, I needed to fuel my body way better than I was doing.

I'll skip a meal because I get so caught up in my day-to-day tasks. My body always alerts me of this mistake by starting to shut down—I feel nauseated, and, not surprisingly, I become grumpy, or "hangry," as some call it.

You don't need to be on a health kick or be a bodybuilder to fuel your body properly. This applies to everyone; we all need fueling every single day. In the book of Daniel, you can read about the food experiment to which Daniel challenged the chief of staff. You see, Daniel did not want to eat the food that the king served because he did not want to defile himself. Daniel asked that they be allowed to eat only vegetables and water for the next ten days; then they could compare themselves to the other men, who ate the king's food. It's no surprise that Daniel and his friends looked healthier and better nourished.

> And at the end of ten days their countenances appeared fairer and fatter in flesh than all the children which did eat the portion of the king's meat. (Daniel 1:15)

I firmly believe there's a twofold reason that they looked healthier. One was that Daniel and his friends honored God by not allowing themselves to be defiled by food the king was serving, so the Lord took care of them. God always honors us when we put Him first, and this is exactly what happened. God used this situation to bring glory to Himself. The other reason is that they ate a very healthy and clean diet; that in itself is conducive to a healthy body and mind. I think this is a good example of doing our part and then allowing God to do the rest.

Have you ever attempted a "Daniel fast"? This consists of a very clean diet, in which you eliminate several categories of food from your everyday eating. There are different opinions on what to eliminate and what you are allowed to eat during a Daniel fast, but the main objective is to grow closer to God through this fasting. You may wonder how fasting can bring us closer to God. Ultimately, eliminating whatever it might be from your life is a sacrifice. This is why we are required to choose something of value to us or needed in our day-to-day lives. Food is a widely used fasting mechanism to grow closer to God, as our bodies need nourishment to survive.

The Daniel fast would be considered a sacrifice for most of us, as it eliminates food that many in society enjoy daily. It's not really about the food, though; it's about the sacrifice. We can ask God to help us eat the food that will bring honor to the bodies He gave us.

Daniel and his friends sacrificed greatly when they rejected the king's food, and the Lord knew that and honored that act of faithfulness. He blessed them with knowledge and skill because of their faithfulness to God. There is something to be said, however, about the way they fed their bodies and how that brought them closer to God. Through discipline and eating the right things, we can work at a full capacity, physically and spiritually.

In the biblical era, they did not have the type of food we have at our fingertips today. They couldn't run to Walmart to grab some snacks for the next day. And there certainly weren't the processed foods that we have readily available to us, making it easier to keep up with our very hectic lives. Even the flour we buy has been processed to a certain degree. Very rarely does a food item go from farm to shelf without human intervention.

In biblical times, they ate food that was grown in their fields, and meat came directly from their own animals. Fruit, vegetables, meat, grains, dairy from their own animals, and honey were some of the everyday foods they consumed.

We quickly understand why they were healthy and had the energy to tackle their very arduous tasks. Some days, we are wiped out from sitting at a desk all day. I fully understand how draining that can be, but perhaps we are so tired because the foods we eat don't nourish us. For example, if our breakfast was a bowl of sugary cereal with our morning coffee, that won't sustain us mentally or physically.

If you have felt tired for a long time, maybe you believe that's how you are supposed to feel. Years ago, that is exactly how I felt about my physical health. Then one day, I thought about how I was feeding my body, and I wondered what God thought about the way I nourished myself.

> So God created man in his own image, in the image of God created he him; male and female created he them. (Genesis 1:27)

I have pondered over the correlation between that scripture and the way we treat our bodies for many years now. I have come to the conclusion that if God created us in His own image, He wants us to take care of it. We know our bodies are only temporal, but while we're here, we should honor His creation.

> Whether therefore ye eat, or drink, or whatsoever ye
> do, do all to the glory of God. (1 Corinthians 10:31)

This scripture tells us that we are to do all things for the glory of God. This encompasses everything that we do in our daily lives, including how we treat the bodies God so lovingly gave us. As Daniel honored God through what he ate, this brought glory to God. Daniel knew to bring glory to God in everything he did.

> I will praise thee; for I am fearfully and wonderfully
> made: marvellous are thy works; and that my soul
> knoweth right well. (Psalm 139:14)

We are fearfully and wonderfully made, just as God intended it to be. It is a shame when we treat our physical bodies like garbage.

We may believe that it doesn't matter because we don't think that we are important, or we don't have enough time, so we feed ourselves garbage—plastic-wrapped food, deep-fried food, processed food, carbonated beverages, and everything that tastes good.

Do you believe that you are important enough to take the time to eat healthy meals? How often have you heard that you are fearfully and wonderfully made? Love yourself the way God loves you. It's constantly used to tell young girls that they are beautiful, no matter what the bullies tell them at school.

The scripture that refers to our being fearfully wonderfully doesn't refer only to the outward appearance; in fact, I would suggest that it may be more about the inward, because if we're honest, we know God cares about that.

And if you believe that what He made is wonderful, then you should take the utmost care of His creation, including nourishing your body. Remember that you put into your body matters. It is a form of self-love to know that you deserve better. How can you be effective in God's kingdom if you are rundown because of your diet?

For years, I was stuck in "slow mode" because of what I was feeding my body. As soon as I decided to care about that area of my life, my mood and energy levels changed drastically. Suddenly, I developed a sense of satisfaction from knowing that I could accomplish more, simply by eating the right food.

God gave us the perfect selection of food that allows our bodies to thrive on this earth. Did I completely stop eating anything that was yummy? Of course not because I also believe that God wants us to enjoy the good things in life—but in moderation. I'm all about moderation. Instead of eating ten cookies, I have two. I don't feel that I'm missing out either. In fact, it's great to enjoy the sweets without feeling sick afterward.

There is also satisfaction that comes with self-control, being aware of your limit and the ability to put it in action. It took time for me to get to this point in my journey with food. My body craved the things I'd been feeding it for years, and it was difficult to apply self-control in the beginning, but it does get easier.

Over time, your body will not crave these things so much, and you may not even have an appetite for them after a while. I'm still surprised when someone offers me fast food and I'm repelled at the thought of it. Instead, my body craves something that is real. If you're traveling on a budget, you might only eat at fast-food chains. By the end of your vacation, you probably cannot wait to get home and have a real meal. That is the state to which your body transitions after dedicated healthy eating over a long time.

You might have heard of *emotional eating*, which is eating to soothe an underlying emotional problem; we either have no idea how to deal with it or don't want to deal with it. Maybe the problem is that you don't love yourself, and because of this, you fill that emptiness inside with food.

Sometimes, we don't know how to help ourselves, or may we not believe there's any point. Nothing could be farther from the truth.

The God who thinks of us, who made us, believes that we are worth it. He left the ninety-nine for us because we are that important. (Read Luke 15:3–7 on how important Jesus believes we are to Him.)

Maybe you think, *I'm too far gone to be helped*. I'm not just talking about food; there is emotional weight attached to all of this. If God believes that you are that valuable—and He does—you should treat yourself as such. Do not insult the Lord by despising the beautiful creation He made—don't forget that He makes no mistakes. Pull down one stronghold after another, and use them as building blocks to reach the full potential that He's had for you this entire time, not only spiritually but in the physical as well.

He made us in His image so that we could go forth and share His love with others, but it starts with us, the all-encompassing us, not only the parts that we have decided are important. Part of our healing is in the physical. We must be ready to do our part. To be fully healed, we must zero in on all parts of our healing that work together for our good.

For this chapter I chose the song "How You See Me Now" by Lydia Laird. It speaks about how God sees us and that we need to see ourselves in the same way.

Listen to this song wherever you are. Pull up the lyrics, pray over them, and allow this truth to permeate your soul.

1. Do you need a physical healing today? Do you need to take a first step in a part to your healing?

2. Similar to the friends of the paralyzed man whom Jesus healed, do you have a friend who needs you to pray for her or him? Do it now, and claim that healing in Jesus's name.

3. What eating habits affect your physical and mental health? Make a list. Tackle each habit, one at a time.

4. List at least three things that you love about yourself and for which you thank God.

5. List three of your attributes that you have a hard time loving. Pray and ask God to help you see them the way He does.

7

PURSUIT OF ACTIVITY

Most of us know that exercise is beneficial, but we often neglect to implement it in our daily lives. Let's look at the definition of *exercise*; then we will redefine the way to look at it as part of our daily lives.

Exercise is defined as "activity requiring physical effort, carried out to sustain or improve health and fitness." Let's examine one word in that definition: *activity*. I believe we need to redefine it to gain a better perspective of what it means to exercise. Hundreds of activities will get our bodies moving as we try to improve our health and fitness. To be physically active does not mean we need to attend a gym five days a week to complete a cross-fit workout. Interestingly, *active* is defined as "engaging or ready to engage in physically energetic pursuits." We should focus on energetic pursuits for physical activity. I adore the word *pursuit* used in the definition of active, for when we pursue something, we are actively setting goals to obtain an end result.

Goals differ from one person to the next; that is what makes life interesting. We each begin our pursuits at a different starting line, and we will meet our goals at different rates. It's important to determine where we should begin our pursuit of activity.

Perhaps the concept of a starting line is holding you back. Maybe you think, *If I need to begin at the bottom, why start at all?* Some of the most successful people began at the bottom and worked their way up to their ultimate goals.

Moses is the perfect example of how a person self-sabotages his walk because of feelings of inadequacy. Moses didn't believe he was the right guy for the job because of his slow speech. Gideon is another great example; he shows us that thinking you're not good enough does not mean you can't carry out the task. Gideon had no confidence in his abilities for the task at hand, but God tells Him otherwise:

> And he said unto him, Oh my Lord, wherewith shall I save Israel? behold, my family is poor in Manasseh, and I am the least in my father's house. And the Lord said unto him, Surely I will be with thee, and thou shalt smite the Midianites as one man. (Judges 6:15–16)

It is a natural reaction for us to belittle our strengths, especially if we've never done that task, or we've had that state of mind for years. We need to push through with God, take that leap of faith, and start wherever we are in our pursuit of activity.

There was a time when I did just that, and it was no small feat for me; it was out of my comfort zone, but I took the plunge. My first fitness class since the beginning of this pregnancy. One foot after another touched the water. The cold temperature of the water permeated my whole body as I slowly submerged my legs. Big inhale and exhale and with much apprehension, my whole body entered the water. I felt so out of place, as I was the only one of my age attending this aquafit class. Aquafit was not new to me; I participated in some sort of water fitness class with most of my babies. This particular fitness program was not for new moms, though, and I had chosen the beginner class. I could sense eyes all over me, most likely wondering what a young person like me was doing in this class, where the average age seemed to be from fifty-five to seventy-five years old. I was the only person there who was in her early thirties.

Several months ago, I enjoyed running two to three times a week. In August, my friend and I completed the Mud Girl Run. I pushed myself to attempt new fitness levels and discovered the real benefits of keeping active.

In November 2019, we found out that we were expecting our fourth child. This pregnancy was very much planned and a huge blessing. As with all of my pregnancies, though, I had morning sickness—all-day sickness is a better description. The inability to eat and hydrate properly affected my energy levels, and all the hormones played with my entire body and mind. Being that ill, there was next to no activity happening. I was in survival mode. I would rejoice daily in things like eating a piece of toast, washing my hair, going grocery shopping, or falling asleep without the horrendous feeling that I was going to be sick. I had three consecutive months with this sense of no control over my body.

But at around the fourth month, I finally started to feel as if I could attempt more than just surviving. That was why I decided to join an Aquafit class; it seemed like a good pursuit of activity. Why the beginner level? My body was no longer used to any fitness routine, and I knew that it would take work to get going again. I actually had no idea that this Aquafit class would be that basic, but I felt like a fish out of water. My first thought was, *What have I done?*

The first moments were very daunting and a little embarrassing. As I lifted my arms and moved my legs, I felt droplets of water hit my face. My body activated in a way that it hadn't in months. Others around me were clearly enjoying this class, and I admired the participants. They were not young, but they had drive and motivation. Suddenly, I realized that, like them, I had drive and motivation to try something new and keep pushing. The feeling of embarrassment and wanting to hide under a rock slowly disappeared with every movement of my body. All those negative feelings were replaced with a sense of accomplishment. I wasn't running a marathon, but I was starting somewhere, and that was where I needed to be.

Isn't that what's important? We judge ourselves for the level where we are or, even worse, where we were five years ago. Maybe we compare ourselves to others and believe we should be at that level by now. It is wrong to do that because someone always will be at a higher or lower level than us. We need to learn to be OK with that. Why should we think that we should be at a different level?

Physically, I needed to begin at level 1. Perhaps I could have started at level 4, but I might have hurt myself or the pregnancy.

In order to begin, you have to go at your own pace, or you will risk slowing down or halting the process. This concept applies not only to physical fitness but to all aspects of life. Start where you are, and move your way up. Feel your leg hit the ground, and continue to lift one leg and one arm at a time. Splash the water, make waves, and let it hit you in the face. This is your journey, and with every movement, you are closer to where you want to be. Be proud of where you are and—most important—where you are going!

Full disclosure—I was not always an advocate for the pursuit of activity, exercise, or physical fitness. Jon, my husband, was my influence in this area. A couple years before I decided to give physical activity a try, he was already deep into the fitness world. He tried cross-fit training, weight lifting, running, and biking. I would tease him about working out because I didn't understand why he felt it was so important. There were times when I would be angry with him that he was so devoted to such a "silly" thing.

I would argue that he was only doing it to build muscle, and he shouldn't make that a top priority in his life. Jon would say that it was not about the muscle; it was about the way he felt after a workout, especially in his mind. The activity was beneficial not only to his body but also for his mental health. I could see that he was happier after exercise, but deep down, I was baffled as to why. I once told him that I didn't need exercise in my life because I was so busy running around, taking care of three children and the house. In my mind, that was enough physical activity for anyone. I didn't need another reason to be more exhausted at the end of the day.

Did it ever get to me when Jon built a mini gym in our basement. I was enraged that were spending money on this stuff. I told him, "You don't need equipment. Rocky Balboa trained without it!"

I now believe that a part of me was jealous of the happiness Jon found in physical activity. *Ouch!* How could I have felt that way toward my husband? We grow every day, and with that, I give myself a little grace. If a friend had expressed these feelings, I would have told her, "You're human. Now that you're aware, you have the capacity to move on." Not too long after I came to the realization that I was jealous, I decided that the sane thing to do was to give exercise a go.

For years, I have battled with total body pain that would come and go. It wasn't debilitating but was an ever-present, nagging kind of pain. It was an ailment that wasn't bothersome enough to go see a doctor, but at the same time, I was sure that something was not right. Jon could tell I was bothered by something and asked about it, but I wouldn't talk about it to anyone except him and then only on days when it was extra annoying. It was another item on my list of things that I just had to live with. This was similar to the thoughts that ran through my mind that I was not an exercise type of person and that just like everyone told me when I was growing up, I was fragile and weaker than others. Exercising was not an activity someone of my caliber should attempt—until one day, I decided that I didn't have anything to lose.

Jon seemed to get so much from it. Who we surround ourselves with is crucial for our personal growth. They will either lift us up or bring us down. Jon had told me from the beginning that I should exercise with him, that it would be an awesome activity to do together. He lifted me up, which allowed me to believe that I could succeed at the pursuit of activity.

I started my pursuit of activity the summer I got a position as an administrative assistant at the Parliament in Ottawa. Employees had access to a well-equipped gym space. It made sense to me; as an assistant, I was sitting all day, so there was no better time for me to start exercising. The feeling that I got from just one session was unreal, and it is truly hard for me to convey how I felt. I'd lived from a place of smallness my whole life, and my eyes were opened to potential I didn't know was inside. Quickly, I saw that the only person stopping me from reaching my goals—whether physical, mental, or spiritual—was me.

I continued with my new exercise regimen. Through my small victories, my desire to grow in this area increased over a long period. Fast-forward two years, and my commitment has only amped up. In fact, it was only after having our fourth child that I implemented it as a regular part of my routine. Being home with Esmée was a joy, but I wanted to make sure that I didn't allow my mind to go down a rabbit hole, like it had so many other times in the past.

Being a stay-at-home parent is a rewarding job, but it was essential for my mental health to care for myself, or I would have lost my mind. Exercise was one of the many practices I put into place to keep myself from becoming depressed.

The pain I'd suffered through for years has dissipated with regular activity! It dawned on me one day as Jon and I were on one of our many walks. Out of nowhere, I asked myself, *When was the last time you were in pain?* I couldn't recall the last time that my body hurt, so I put two and two together. It was not just by chance that the pain had disappeared. I know this because as soon as I take a break from exercising for a few days or more, the pain creeps back in with a vengeance. No coincidence in this situation. Only when my body stops moving does pain start to take hold.

Movement is essential for full-body functional health. Your body was not built to sit around and not use it to the full capacity that God intended. There is a reason that He gave us the ability to move every muscle; everything has been planned to the last detail.

Think on this: what happens when you hurt a muscle or a ligament, maybe one that you didn't know existed? You probably realize that you need that muscle to function for other things to work properly.

All things work together for our good, planned by God, and this applies to our bodies. If one part doesn't operate at full capacity, then the rest will overcompensate, which will cause the whole to break down over time.

We are told that our bodies are temples of the Holy Spirit and that we are to glorify God in our bodies.

> Or do you not know that your body is the temple of the Holy Spirit who is in you, whom you have from God, and you are not your own? For you were bought at a price; therefore glorify God in your body and in your spirit, which are God's. (1 Corinthians 6:19–20)

Not only is God telling us to glorify Him in our bodies but that we were bought with a price. Our freedom was purchased with the greatest sacrifice ever known, and if we are to glorify God on earth, then we must do so in the body too. We are walking, living, and breathing testaments for each person we encounter on our individual journeys. It's about allowing God to bring us to levels we never thought possible. As we are not our own, we must carefully protect what was given to us. When you borrow an item from a friend, you probably take more care with it than with items that belong to you. You want to return the item in the same condition you received it and sometimes even better.

Unfortunately, life is full of hardships, which makes it impossible to return your body in better shape than the way it arrived. But it is not in vain to strive for a healthy and functional body. There may be extenuating circumstances, and you may not be able to do what everyone else can, but you certainly can give it your all. God will give you the full strength you need to continue. Remember, though, not to compare yourself with others; that is a dangerous road to embark on.

How can we push through our human weaknesses and stop ourselves from succumbing to our fleshly desires? The flesh is weak; this we know from experience and from scripture. It is only through the Spirit that we gain our strength—not our own but God's. John 14:16–17 tells us where our help comes from:

> And I will pray the father and He will give you another Helper, that He may abide with you forever - the spirit of truth, whom the world cannot receive, because it neither sees Him nor knows Him; but you know Him, for He dwells with you and will be in you.

Our bodies are temples of the Holy Spirit. This scripture ties with 1 Corinthians 6:19–20, in that if we are the temple of the Holy Spirit, then He abides in us; one purpose for that is to be our helper. The Greek word for abide is *meno*, which means to remain, stay, endure, or inhabit. The Spirit in us is here to stay, helping us endure and overcome the tribulations of this world by inhabiting our very bodies.

The Spirit is an important aid in our spiritual lives, and we should hold on to that truth. The Spirit, however, also should be our help in our physical walk on this earth. If we are not strong in our bodies, then it will be extremely difficult for us to endure the trials that life throws at us. Making our tests, which become our testimonies, seem impossible.

I find it intriguing that the Greek definition for *abide* includes the word *endure*. Seems to me that this is proof that the Spirit was meant to help us endure all things. To *endure* is to have the capacity to walk through trials, feeling the pressure and perhaps the desire to quit, but we press on, knowing that the Spirit abides in us and that we are not alone. The Spirit is our champion, every step of the way.

More often than not, our flesh will push back in the pursuit of activity, as our natural fleshly desire is to sit back and relax, especially in our hectic lives. We must refrain from falling into the trap of complacency, including in our walk toward physical health. It's easier to sit down after dinner than to push ourselves to take a walk. One hour of extra sleep sounds much more enjoyable than rising with the birds to get active. We may have a million excuses not pursue daily activity—we're too busy with the kids, or our jobs won't allow for that kind of time.

It could very well be that you *are* too busy, but only you can make a lifestyle change. The pursuit of activity for physical health is a choice you need to make every day. In everything you do—in any type of activity—your first step should be with God by your side. He needs to be at the center of it all.

> And whatsoever ye do in word or deed, do all in the name of the Lord Jesus, giving thanks to God and the Father by him. (Colossians 3:17)

If God is at the center of all we do, then He will direct our paths and give us the strength we need to keep going. When I pursue any physical activity, there is a constant prayer in my heart, asking Him to provide the strength required to complete the task and whatever the day ahead may bring. During my daily activity, I frequently praise and thank Him for my ability to be active. I am very aware that not everyone is able to tackle these exercises on a regular basis.

We should not forget where our strength comes from. God is the source of our strength, and we are only as strong as we allow Him to work in our lives. Our circumstances tend to dictate how we see ourselves and how strong we believe we are. If we remember where our strength comes from, then we will know that whatever lies in front of us is already overcome through Him.

Before I knew where my strength came from, I believed the lie whispered in my ear for years: *You are weak.* Now, when I feel the adrenaline rush from a workout, there is overwhelming thankfulness in my spirit through the knowledge and awareness that God has given me this opportunity. Every time my foot hits the ground and lifts back up on a run, I know who has given me this privilege. Some days, a workout doesn't happen, whether for physical or mental health reasons. I still praise God for the gift of life, the sunrise that morning, and my feet hitting the ground as I climbed out of bed. If all I can do that day is simply function, then I can thank Him for the strength to do that, and every day is a new day filled with new mercies.

Lamentations 3:22–23 reminds of God's daily faithfulness, on which we can depend:

> It is of the Lord's mercies that we are not consumed, because his compassions fail not. They are new every morning: great is thy faithfulness.

Perhaps you think that working out is not your thing. Someone says *exercise*, and you freeze. Discomfort with fear overcomes your mind because when you think about physical activity, you see marathons, heavy-duty weights, or attending a gym religiously. Maybe you're right that those types of physical activity will never be your cup of tea, but everyone needs to be active.

Jesus always required action for a healing or promise. Take a look at the Israelites, walking through the wilderness. He did not magically swoop them up and—voila—they found themselves in the promised land. No, they had a destination to walk toward. It took far longer than He intended, but they had their part to play to receive their promise.

Could He have made the ark appear for Noah and his family? Of course, but He asked Noah to build the ark and gave him the instructions for it. The paralyzed man was asked to pick up his bed and walk—he was asked to have enough faith to get up and walk. The woman with the issue of blood fought her way to touch the hem of His garment; she had to make her way to Jesus for her healing. When He healed the ten lepers, they were asked to show themselves to the priests—again, another action to be taken for a healing. As they walked, their healing was fulfilled.

When we take action and have enough faith to walk toward our healing, God walks with us, no questions asked. In these lessons, we also see that if He asks us to do something, He will tell us what is required. *Faith* is to believe in the unseen, and once we have that, He will guide us toward our destination. He will not require big faith from us and then allow us to make mistake after mistake.

Listen. He is telling you what is asked of you. Faith is not simply believing but the ability to gird your loins and take the next step. Walk, if that is all your body will allow you to do, even if you start with only twice a week. Work your way up from twice a week to three as you praise and thank Him for the victory. Watch as you grow stronger, not only in your body but also in Him, knowing that He is your daily and ultimate strength.

Maybe you want to try yoga. Start with the beginner class or prenatal class, even if you're not pregnant. Don't be ashamed of where you are because God certainly isn't. Has it been so hard that simply climbing the stairs once a day is a struggle? Climb the stairs two times with the utmost care and caution, but do it and be proud. As you do this, listen to "This Could Change Everything" by Francesca Battistelli, and allow yourself to believe that this is your moment.

Start the pursuit of activity today, whatever that means for you. Be consumed with the idea that physical freedom is not just for others and that the all-powerful God you serve wants you to glorify Him in your body by reaching the full potential He's already set aside for you. Walk, run, dance, skip, or crawl toward it, knowing that you deserve a healthy body and that He will strengthen you with each step.

1. Everyone has a secret ambition that they never speak about. What physical activity have you always wanted to try, but you chose to believe you couldn't do it?

2. Take that ambition and pursue it actively. Lay out the steps you will need to accomplish this goal. At which level will you need to start to be successful?

3. What are the lies that constantly circle in your mind in regard to physical activity? Acknowledge them; then pray for the strength to rebuke them, right now and in the future.

4. Knowing that your flesh is weak, from where does your strength need to constantly come? What scripture promises us that God will forever abide in us and be our helper?

8

BE A GILMORE GIRL

In addition to feeding and moving our bodies, it's important to rest our bodies. For some, this may be a hard thing to do; it seems that something always needs to be done. Others may say they already know the importance of rest, but knowing that rest is beneficial does not mean they practice it. Without a doubt, we need to normalize resting so that we no longer feel guilty about resting.

I often hear people say they take time to rest, but that's followed by guilt-filled shame, as they believe they should have accomplished a task instead. When their allotted rest time is over, they work double time to catch up on all the things they think they should have done. Essentially, they punish themselves for taking time to rest, which makes absolutely no sense because rest is a need for every human on this earth.

We don't get to skip rest and hope for the best, which is what most of us do, but then we crash and burn. Burnout, depression, anxiety, and insomnia are just some of the side effects of no rest. Why are depression and anxiety listed as side effects? Because, as you might remember, the mind, body, and soul are interrelated. Each affects the other as a whole. An exhausted body is more prone to suffer from depression and anxiety. The body gets tired and becomes unable to support itself properly. It becomes a drain on the other areas of functionality until it simply cannot sustain the rhythm we've maintained for so long.

Why do we punish ourselves for taking much-needed rest time? Before the pandemic, we were always busy doing something, whether work-related or socially. The popular vibe was that if we were not busy, then our lives must not be fulfilling, or perhaps there was something wrong with us. Of course, not everyone had this mentality, but a large percent of the population sure did. This idea is similar to "keeping up with the Joneses" but specifically focusing on how busy we are. So-and-so ran errands, had company over for lunch, cleaned her home in the afternoon, and was making dessert for dinner plans later. She also found the time to work out, do the laundry, send work emails, prep for responsibilities at church on Sunday, and take the dog for a walk. These commitments were done in one day because occupying each and every single minute of her day was crucial. Her success was measured by how much you were able to physically conquer in a day.

Not many of us talk about how a person might feel at the end of a day like that. We don't see this person crash on her bed, exhausted, wishing she had enough willpower to take some rest for herself, nor do we see the tears that were streaming down her face as she folded the laundry because she had no idea how she would get through the rest of the day. We are unaware of the pain in her body from the intense physical labor to which she's subjected herself, with no room for rest.

Then the pandemic hit, and we went from filling our schedules to staying home and being creative with all that free time. In the blink of an eye, we went from one extreme to the other. For some, this was a major shock to their everyday lives, whereas others quickly fell seamlessly into this new beat. As time went on, people accepted this new way of life and—dare I say it?—enjoyed their new freedom. The social contracts that the everyday life used to hold became a thing of the past.

Please don't misunderstand me; I firmly believe that we human beings require social interaction. We were never meant to be isolated and alone for long periods. The pandemic, however, brought a new revelation with regard to what we thought was important. Many of us realized that very little of the hustle and bustle was essential to our happiness and that our physical sprint each day kept us from seeing life's wonderful moments.

When my children were really young, I would run myself ragged at home while also caring for them, physically demanding my body to perform in ways that it was not made to do. By the end of the day, I was an empty shell, and Jon had to deal with the "mood." In my mind, I believed it was possible to do all the chores and more in one day. At the workplace, I pushed myself to complete every task in one day, essentially setting impossible standards for myself.

It doesn't matter which walk we are on. We seem to think we have superpowers—until our bodies fail us and give us a reality check. Our poor bodies tried to tell us, with little signs here and there, whispering to us that it cannot go on this way much longer. But like the check-engine light that flashes in our cars, sometimes we just ignore it, hoping it will hold out a little longer.

From my experience, I can tell you that it is never good when my body is forced to halt all operations. In fact, when my body reaches a certain level of exhaustion, my mind starts to run wild, causing anxiety. In recent years, I've noticed my anxiety level is a signal to me that I'm doing too much without enough rest. In retrospect, it's a blessing to see the signs of physical exhaustion—without those signs, I'm apt to keep pushing until my body crashes and burns.

Another telltale sign for me is my mood level. I tend to become more grumpy and less present in the moment. It's sort of a brain fog from overexertion. All the tasks and life around me seem to lump together as one, and I lose the ability to compartmentalize what needs to be done. When I lose that ability, my emotions are no longer my own.

Control of the mind becomes increasingly difficult with the

more weight you add to your already full plate. Remember—and I can't stress this enough—that the mind is connected to the body, and one impacts the other in almost everything you do.

The body, of course, is only temporal, while we are here on earth. It was never meant to last forever and is weak on its own. When we know we are weak without God, then we know where to go to find our strength and rest. This, however, does not mean that we shouldn't take care of our bodies. God knew that our bodies would need rest. Genesis 2:2–3 tells us that even God took a day of rest:

> And on the seventh day God ended his work which
> he had made; and he rested on the seventh day from
> all his work which he had made. And God blessed
> the seventh day, and sanctified it: because that in it
> he had rested from all his work which God created
> and made.

One of the many takeaways from this particular scripture is that the type of rest God knows we need is not only for the body. We must reach a spiritual rest, which, not surprisingly, will restore us in mind, body, and soul. From the beginning, God knew that we would have to work hard to sustain ourselves during our time on earth. Most importantly, being the sovereign God that He is, He also knew that we would need rest from our hard labor. The Sabbath wasn't given to us because God was weary or needed rest; it was made for humans.

> And he said to them, The sabbath was made for
> man, not man for sabbath. (Mark 2:27)

Think about it: God has given us the permission—not only permitted, but He has told us explicitly to rest in Him. We have no reason to feel guilty about taking the time to rest. How can we argue with a God who created it all in seven days and then took time to rest, just so we would do the same. Our work is certainly not more important than His, and still, He felt it essential to rest.

You might be wondering about the title of this chapter, "Be a Gilmore Girl." First, you need to know that my all-time favorite show is *Gilmore Girls*; in fact, I watch this show just to rest. It's the story of a mom and daughter who are extremely close—really more like best friends than parent and child. Lorelai, the mother, works arduously to build a successful life while raising her teenage daughter, Rory. I find it fabulous that when they rest, there is a no-nonsense vibe about it—no guilt attached to it, simply living their best lives.

I'm not saying we should rest in the same way that Lorelai and Rory go about it, but what if we were bold enough to rest without guilt attached. On a Friday night after a long week, the Gilmore girls will have picked a movie or two, which they will watch while enjoying their favorite junk foods. They allow time to slow down in their daily lives. Our society would have a person feeling guilty about relaxing instead of cleaning the house or catching up on the laundry. Why, though? Life is short, and as blessed people, there is nothing wrong with relaxing after a long week of work.

In one episode of *Gilmore Girls*, Rory wakes Lorelai excruciatingly early one Saturday. The conversation goes as follows:

Lorelai: Rory, my heart, today is Saturday, the day of rest!

Rory: Sunday's the day of rest.

Lorelai: No, Saturday's the day of pre-rest.

Rory: Pre-rest?

Lorelai: Yeah, so that way when you actually get to Sunday, you're rested enough to enjoy your rest.

Rory: That makes absolutely no sense.

Lorelai: That's because it's six o'clock on Saturday morning!

It was meant to be a funny conversation, but there is a profound truth in the statement about "pre-rest." We have the capability to not completely come to a stop but still achieve a slower pace than usual.

We may feel that the weekend is never long enough and that we don't feel rested, come Monday. Maybe that's because there was no pre-rest involved in our routines—a slow-down button, a downshift in gears as we prepare to stop. When we come to our day of rest, we haven't allowed for room to decompress, and it's a shock to the body. Come Monday, the body is not ready to get going. Mind and body both think, *Wait—what? I was just getting to a place of rest.*

In order to understand what the word *rest* means, I researched the Greek meaning, which includes a couple of words that stood out to me: intermission and cessation. An *intermission* is a pause or break from an activity or task. This specific word always triggers a memory I have when Jon took me to *The Nutcracker.* It was my very first ballet, a long-awaited bucket list item. I became so excited about this event that I felt ill. As we were sitting in the theater, waiting for the show to start, I felt my emotions slowly get the best of me. To say I was disappointed by my lack of control of my emotions would be an understatement. Jon was so gracious, as he always is, and he did whatever he could to help me. I was very aware that he was disappointed too because he'd been excited to give me this surprise.

As you might imagine, I was thankful when the intermission arrived. This gave me a chance to step out, get some air, and get my bearings. A moment to pause was just what I needed, along with a supportive husband. We'd been together long enough for him to know that this was not out of the ordinary for me.

After the intermission, I was able to sit down and enjoy the second half of the show. Now, when I hear the word *intermission,* my mind goes back to that moment in time—an instant in my life when I needed a pause more than ever.

There was no question in God's mind when He decided that we would need intermissions in our lives. But sometimes, we need cessation—to cease what we are doing altogether, which is why I think that both intermission and cessation perfectly describe the meaning of rest. These two words can be used interchangeably when we refer to rest in our bodies, minds, and souls. An intermission will not be enough for us at times, depending on the season we are in. There will be a time when we will have to cease whatever activity, task, or life hurdle is in front of us. It would be wise to learn to read our bodies so that we know which type of rest to take.

As I was writing this book, I had to lay down something to fully focus on the task. With the Ladies Conference coming up, I'd have to decide whether or not I would be a vendor at the event. As I've mentioned, it's my favorite event of the year, and I make and sell headbands at it. I knew that it would be a struggle to handle both the event and writing, so I'd have to choose between being overwhelmed or ceasing something, just for a season. From past experiences with overfilling my plate, I decided not to sell my headbands at Ladies Conference. I would enjoy the conference to the full extent and get some writing done, if time permitted. It felt rewarding to have the ability to say no and to feel rested in my body before attending. Normally, I'd run myself to the point that my whole body ached from the extreme push of work it took to prepare for such an event. How liberating it was to no longer allow the pressure to perform a certain way, as society so often dictates.

Being in tune with God allows us to hear His whispers of rest, and being confident that is exactly what He wants for us. There is healing within the rest that God can give us in our bodies, minds, and souls. Like most lessons in life, I learned this the hard way through falling more times than I can count. As I've mentioned, the way I was brought up was not conducive to any type of rest.

Our childhoods deeply affect the persons we later become in life, whether giving us healthy or unhealthy habits. Through no fault of my parents, our household had a military vibe, which means that rest was for the weak—if you weren't doing something, then you were a failure. The reason I do not blame my parents is that they were brought up this way. They didn't know anything different because they had always done things that way. I remember the feeling of sitting on my bed, not doing anything, but feeling apprehensive of the wrath that would soon enter my room, asking me what I was doing, or saying, "Surely there are chores or homework you could be completing."

I carried this well into my adult years and believed that this was the way of all families. Only a few years ago did God show me that this mentality was not His will for me or anyone. My hustle-hard state of being was not only preventing me from attaining His will, but it was also unwholesome for me and my family. As God began to show me the error in my ways, I also saw that I was doing this to my own children. Out of nowhere, I would get in a frenzy about the things that needed to be done and would shout orders to those I loved most.

It took me a long time to write the previous sentence, and I almost wanted to omit it. I dislike the fact that I acted in such a manner at any point in my life. In order to truly shine my testimony, however, you must know the good, bad, and ugly, if only to show you that God can change anyone.

The healing I found in rest is not comparable to anything I've ever experienced. Rest of the body is and always will be a component that must be reached to be healed. As I gave myself permission to be a "Gilmore girl," my healing was elevated to a whole new level. When I speak of resting the body, I don't mean that I sit around all day watching movies. It's that I allowed myself to pick up a book, read a devotion, sit outside in the sun, take a bath, or even grab a quick nap. All things work together for good, and as I did these restful things, my mind and soul were also nourished. Feeding one part of the whole usually results in a domino effect that produces fruit in other areas of our lives.

Will there be times in your life when you need to lie down and do absolutely nothing? Yes, of course, and that is OK. It's better to allow yourself one or two days of *dolce far niente* than to burn out and need months of rest to heal a very broken self.

It is vain for you to rise up early, to sit up late, to
eat the bread of sorrows: for so he giveth his beloved
sleep. (Psalm 127:2)

Let's establish that you are God's beloved, a child of God. His
love cannot be compared to human affection; it is far greater than
that. To be His beloved is to be deeply loved by God, so much that
He wants you to get rest. Christy Nockels wrote a book called *The
Life You Long For. Learning to Live from a Heart of Rest,* an excellent
read that goes in depth about being God's beloved. I've read it once
and will read it again—it's that good. She says,

Sometimes choosing a heart of rest involves being
honest with ourselves and honest about our agendas,
recognizing that we actually can't and don't have
to do it all. When we invite Jesus to live His life
through us, we find ourselves on His grace-paved
path, where His way of doing life is easy and His
burden is light.

To live from a heart rest allows for a state of being that will flow
to the body, mind, and soul. Our agendas, as Christy Nockels writes,
are jammed packed, if we are honest with ourselves. We must take a
look at our agendas, and be honest with ourselves. What needs to be
done, and what is just extra? We cannot do it all, and Jesus certainly
never expected us to do it all. That is part of the reason why we are
all different, offering unique gifts given to us by God. We were not
meant to do it all; others are capable and perhaps more gifted in a
certain area. When we attempt to be everything to everyone, we
slowly start to spiral, causing stress on ourselves, which those around
us can feel. We need to learn how to allow others to take over some
areas in our lives to which we cling. Jesus wants us to let go and to
perhaps allow someone else to bloom.

Stress affects the body; it places a weight on us—an invisible but present force weighing us down—that physically affects us. The saying, "I feel like a weight has been lifted off my shoulders" is literal in its relation to the physical body. We may not be able to see the weight of the stress we're carrying, but it is there. If we would place the weight down and allow Jesus to pick it up for us, we could rest in His arms while He carries us through what might feel impossible.

He has done this for me many times, carrying me through the trials and expectations of each day. As I tried to complete my diploma in the law clerk program in Ottawa, while taking care of my family of three, I quickly became overwhelmed. Not only was I going to school as a young mom, but certain plans for childcare did not pan out like we had planned.

As God always does, He took care of the situation. Wonderful friends offered to watch Cohen, who was only about three years old, making it possible for me to attend my classes. People asked me how I was able to go to school full time with a family to care for. That was a great question, as I often felt like I was making it by the skin of my teeth. Most often, when we are in the thick of it, the ability to clearly see where our strength comes from is blurred. We may only have the strength to put one foot in front of the other some days, so we fail to see that we did make it through each day. We are focused on our distress and not on the small victories. There are times when we are not even walking but are carried by God. During what felt like a balancing act that was coming close to crumbling, I have no doubt that He carried me on many of those days.

As you give yourself permission to enter God's rest, play the song "Rest" by Kari Jobe. Your relationship with God will flourish as you rest with Him. He never leaves you, dear friend. When you feel like He has, perhaps He is carrying you. I know that He has carried me countless times, allowing me to rest in His arms. Are you entering into His rest, or do you jump out of His arms when you see another "task," only to find yourself more exhausted? Physical rest is extremely important. Stop guilt-tripping yourself every time you enter into His rest. To give Him everything you have for the kingdom, you will also need rest that is given to you, should you choose to lay down your agenda and physically stop.

Again, this is a daily healing that you must accept and work toward, as your healing will be made whole only with every piece fitting together. Enjoy the life He greatly sacrificed for you to have. Don't waste it in trying to fulfill the things that can wait—most things can wait, if you really think about it. I've heard that if we were to die tomorrow, a replacement would be found for our positions within a week's time. Keep in mind, though, that according to God, there is no replacement for each of us. We are each uniquely made for His purpose. In order to fulfill His purpose, we must learn how to rest in His presence.

Work hard. Pray hard. Rest hard.

1. Think about how much time you allow for rest in any given week. Do you need to adjust your schedule to allow yourself to enter into the rest that you need?

2. Are there commitments that you need to release from your life?

3. What activities or hobbies would you like to start doing in your time off? If you haven't a clue, research "hobbies" on the internet, and see if anything sparks your interest.

4. Does the song "Rest" by Kari Jobe speak to you? Does it inspire you to enter into God's rest?

9

PERFECT POSTURE

As we have determined, there are endless physical ramifications from stress. Toxic relationships can cause severe physical ailments, even if you are not aware of it, especially if you are in a toxic relationship. Toxic relationships suck you dry, physically, emotionally, mentally, and spiritually. I believe that Christians are more susceptible to it because we believe that we are to love everyone; we are called to love just as God loves us.

It is possible, however, to love someone and not be slowly poisoned by his or her bad behavior.

As an extremely sensitive person, I feel everything on a deep level. If I'm in a room where anger, hate, anxiety, suffering, or depression are present, I will feel all these emotions within me. Empathy can be a wonderful quality, except when you do not know how to control it. I don't believe that anyone is a stranger to toxic relationships; at some point, we've all had some encounter with this type of person. Often, we hold on longer than we should, believing that we can change the person. We may believe that *we* are the problem, and we should change or be a better person.

Your healing will come to a grinding halt when you are dealing with a toxic relationship. These relationships will have you believe something about yourself that is not true. You'll be distracted on an entirely other level, blind to what is happening around you.

Proverbs 4:23 says it is your job to guard your heart: "Keep thy heart with all diligence; for out of it are the issues of life." What does it mean to keep your heart? You need to protect your heart from the things that come to disturb it and throw it off balance. To protect your heart, you need to be careful what or who you allow into your life.

I am no stranger to toxic relationships. In fact, my experience comes from within my family, which makes it so much more difficult. I've had to make some very heart-wrenching but necessary decisions so that I could be a whole and functional human being. When we are exposed to toxic relationships, our minds produce toxic thoughts, which is usually followed by physical illness. Toxic relationships are like poison in the physical body. For years, I did my best to maintain these relationships because there was no other choice. When my physical and mental health was affected, however, I had to put a stop to them.

Have you ever walked into a room and felt a heavy presence that you did not feel before entering? Perhaps you have picked up the phone, and then your insides turn upside down when you find out who is calling. Sometimes being in the same home as someone with erratic behavior will have you in a constant state of mental alertness. Every time you are around such a person, you feel you must walk on eggshells so you don't set the bomb off with a simple comment. If you do not act a certain way, then you are in for a treat, as according to the person, that is the right way. You may have the feeling that you are being manipulated into being someone you are not.

I've been yelled at because of the hat I was wearing. One beautiful summer day, my family and I arrived at our destination. I was wearing a beautiful, classy white sunhat. I felt so great and elegant wearing it. Funny how a silly piece of clothing or accessory can make us feel that way, but I just felt pretty. Upon our arrival, someone said to me, disapprovingly, "Where did you get that hat?"

I could tell that this person hated the way I looked in my hat, but I didn't know why. As the day went on, I heard the same person make more snide remarks about my hat. It became increasingly clear that my hat was causing some kind of disturbance in this person's life.

The next day was my birthday, and I had the brilliant idea of going to a restaurant so that everyone could relax, with no dishes to be done. Mistake of mistakes—had I known it would cause so much drama, a bowl of cereal would have made me happy. Things did not go well from that point on. I was yelled at and accused of many things, and there were derogatory comments about the hat. I just wanted to be me! What was wrong with me, that I couldn't just be myself?

This one instance is simply the tip of the iceberg. I cannot even count the number of times I've been yelled at, manipulated, and made to feel small, worthless, and not enough. I had a constant ill feeling in my stomach whenever I was around this person, as I never knew what to expect. In one second, this person would be fine; in the next, it was as I had caused a brutal wrong. The worst experience was when this person would call and talk with me as if nothing had happened. How was it OK for a person to have that type of power in my life? I felt like I'd lost my marbles—had I imagined what had occurred?

When I was walking, I would look down because that is where I thought I deserved to be. The constant verbal abuse was getting to me physically. I felt like I was not worthy of anything, and if I keep my head down, it would make me a harder target—because I felt like a target, being mocked or constantly told what was wrong with me as a person.

This kind of treatment doesn't affect only one relationship in your life; it transfers over into every aspect of life. It is scientifically proven that our posture has a direct correlation with our physical and mental health. Someone who is depressed or has low self-esteem is more apt to slump due to his or her mental state. Bad posture also affects our physical health, so it is a vicious circle. The long-term physical impact from slouching is surprising—it can lead to poor blood and oxygen flow throughout the body.

Try it right now. Are you sitting in a slouched position? Sit up straight, and then take a few deep breaths. You will feel that the air flow is much easier. Consistent slouching also can cause heartburn or acid reflux. The problem starts in the mind but ends up directly affecting the body.

When you are subject to a toxic relationship, one common reaction is to hide how you feel. If you have attempted to voice your feelings but have been shut down many times and are told to stop being dramatic, it's normal to stop trying to be heard. Take heart. I understand how frustrating it is to speak with this type of person. Over time, you push your emotions deep down inside, hoping they will just go away. You don't know what to do, and it's better not to deal with the sadness anymore.

This is not reality; we cannot push our emotions to the curb. The reality is that sadness, rejection, anger, and any other emotions you feel are still there. You are simply ignoring them. Unfortunately, you can ignore something only for so long before it becomes a big problem. A roof that has a slow leak might not seem like a huge deal, but if ignored, that slow drip will cause more damage than if you had dealt with it when the problem arose.

In our current home, there was a slow leak within the window and the roof. We had no idea—until the drywall gave out in our son's room one morning. This leak was miniscule, and the window company had it fixed within ten minutes, but the damage caused on the inside was unbelievable, given the size of the hole. Because we didn't know about it, water had accumulated in the wood and drywall until it couldn't hold anymore.

You will not be able to hold in those emotions forever. You may think, *I've got this*, and it might be that you do for the moment. But what are the toxic relationships keeping you from? Proverbs 22:24–25 gives us insight about what might happen if we choose to continue in toxic relationships:

> Make no friendship with a man given to anger, nor
> go with a wrathful man, lest you learn his ways and
> entangle yourself in a snare.

Toxic relationships do not produce the fruits of the Spirit. They are based on anger, manipulation, a condescending nature, stress, and control, and these relationships are in no way fruitful. Should we choose to travel down this path with a toxic person, we will eventually acquire some of that person's personality traits. Without being aware of our change, we will treat others in the way that we are being treated.

You may be dealing with physical abuse in addition to verbal abuse. This is no joke, and it's certainly not a trait you want to pass on to those around you. Realize that the decision to deal with these relationships is not only for you but for those around you who are watching for guidance.

The definition of a *mentor* is an experienced and trusted adviser. In some capacity, we each will be a mentor to someone, whether to our children, grandchildren, friend, or niece or nephew. This could be anyone who looks to us for advice or guidance in any area of their lives. We want to be sure that they have solid character traits to model within their own lives. It rarely is just about us; there is always a bigger purpose behind everything. We were given salvation not only for ourselves but to be witnesses to others around us. How can we do that if we allow toxic relationships to destroy what we know to be right?

It is beneficial to healing that we are open and speak about the pain behind these relationships. As we do this, our souls open up to healing, and we learn things of which we were completely unaware. Through opening up, we may learn what really hurts us and why we function in a certain way. A superficial cut heals faster when it is left to air out and dry .

You might not be able to do that right away with a deep wound, the Band-Aid protects the wound from the harsh elements. Soon, though, the wound will be ready to face the elements and will heal quicker because you gave it a chance to open up and breathe.

Closing up is how you invite physical ailments, anxiety, and depression into your life. You are not dealing with your emotions, and you probably are not welcoming any help from those around you. How can a friend or family member help you if you don't voice what you're going through? Maybe you don't want to be that person who constantly laments about his or her situation, but there is a distinct difference between being a martyr and being open enough to accept help when needed.

Before healing was a daily ritual in my life, I believed that external help was not necessary. I'd made it this far on my own; surely I could go the rest of the way, even if that meant crawling. The act of crawling is OK and is often necessary in our trials, but every now and then, we need someone to pick us up for some respite. Babies crawl for much of their day within their homes—that's how they learn—but you would never let a baby crawl on a strenuous hike. So how is it different for you as you try to navigate your storm? Sometimes, the journey is too long to crawl to the finish line; you need a helping hand along the way.

We have the ability to choose how we deal with and react to the toxic relationships in our lives. We all have a breaking point, and we need to decide what our responses will be to certain people. Some of us will hit rock bottom before we realize that things need to change. My rock bottom was when the relationship caused me to wonder how much my life was worth. I was destroyed and beaten down by verbal abuse and constant rejection, and I wondered if it was worth it to stick around. This toxic person had always been my rock and the one person who should have loved me, no matter what. As you might imagine, the fall of that relationship broke me in a way I'd never thought possible.

I love plants, flowers, and all things that grow into something beautiful. There is something miraculous in seeing a plant grow from a tiny seed and transform. Before I had kids, I completed my degree in floral design. (It really is a thing.) I studied the names of all the flowers and plants that are most commonly stocked in a flower shop. I learned how to create beautiful floral arrangements. My work space would be a complete disaster after I finished, but the arrangement would be gorgeous.

I segued from floral design to the law clerk program when our third child was about three years old, but that was mostly for practical reasons. I figured a job with a pension and that was easier on my body was wise. My love for plants and flowers never diminished, though. It shouldn't be surprising that I decided to read a book called *Lessons from Plants* by Brenda L. Montgomery. This book is chock-full of life lessons from the perspective of a plant's purpose and life-surviving techniques.

As I was reading one of the chapters, I realized how much it related to the process of deciding what to do with toxicity in our lives. Plants go through a special process called the "detection, judgment, decision paradigm." A plant has the ability to detect environmental cues through sensors, including light, temperature, and moisture. A plant utilizes these sensors so it can adapt its response to surrounding environmental factors. The adapted responses a plant puts into place are planning, modulating growth, and warding off danger.

Plants are budget-conscious in regard to their energy efficiency and investment. They tend avoid competition when they can and decide how to spend their energy. As they learn about the environment around them, they choose to either confront and compete, collaborate, tolerate, or avoid altogether. Plants can be resilient in very unfavorable environments.

When there is rivalry for light, a plant will enter into *shade-avoidance behavior*. This is the activation of growth-promoting hormones that send signals to the stems, telling them to elongate. Why? Because if the stems elongate, they can "win" the battle for light. A shade-tolerant plant may choose to tolerate these conditions, as it is better equipped to survive in low-light conditions.

Plants also have the ability to attract beneficial environmental factors or to repel predators through the release of compounds in the air. For example, a corn plant that is attacked by a moth larva has the power to release a chemical that will attract a parasitic wasp. This is ingenious—the wasp will arrive and feed on the larva, preventing any further damage to the plant. The chemical released has another purpose—as a precautionary defense mechanism. The plant alerts its neighbors of potential danger.

How fascinating is it that plants have options for survival, depending on their environment. Based on their genetic makeup, some are able to tolerate certain conditions better than others. No matter what a plant decides to implement, however, the end goal is always survival and to flourish.

A plant is budget-conscious regarding the energy it expends, and we should mimic this same practice. Deciding where our energy is spent allows us to seriously examine the circumstances and people we allow in our lives. When we intentionally choose where to put our energy, everything is put into perspective on levels of importance and value. We then will seek relationships and lifestyles that nourish our energy levels, instead of choosing to engage in energy-leaching customs and people.

Maybe you have already tried to disperse your energy in the right places and have limited the amount of time you spend with toxic people. Perhaps you feel like the plant that has a rivalry for light, and you constantly feel as if you need to compete and elongate your stems to reach the light you need to thrive. You're exhausted from the never-ending battle between energy efficiency and fighting for survival. Every time you get one step ahead, that relationship throws another curveball, and you are back in survival mode. *Weary* doesn't begin to describe how you feel from constantly trying to grow, just for survival. You can feel your body starting to fail you with each push forward.

Growing is part of life that is entirely different from being forced to grow for survival. You may be painfully aware that even with all your efforts to conserve energy, you will not be able to keep on like this forever. This is where it becomes extremely difficult to make the next decision. You know, deep down, that the next step is crucial for your physical, mental, and spiritual health, but you're also conscious that no matter how you do it, there is always pain tied with the following phase.

Excruciatingly painful resolve is often necessary to cut certain relationships out of your life. After years of trying to have a somewhat normal relationship, which always seemed to fail, there is no other solution for your survival—and even more important, for your healing. Similar to the plant that releases chemicals to prevent further damage, you need to assess how much more damage you are able to take. I said *able* instead of *willing* because there is a difference.

You might be *willing* to take a few more hits, but the question is, is your body *able* to endure more upper cuts, jabs, left hooks, and gut-wrenching hurt. It takes practice to know when to release that chemical compound for survival. With time, you will be able to discern when someone or something is a drain on your life. Like plants, you will pick up on environmental cues that tell you what needs to be done. I don't believe it ever gets easy to make this kind of decision, but you will learn that it is in your best interest. The action is difficult, but the outcome always leads to healing.

As I rehashed my decision to cut that toxic relationship out of my life, I asked the same questions: Did I make the right decision? Should I have tried harder to make it work? Does the person think of me and miss me? But then I looked at how far I'd come since that difficult decision. That was part of my healing process, and because of it, I grew by leaps and bounds in ways that I never imagined possible.

The old me walked with a slouch as I tried to physically hide myself; I truly believed I was not worth the fight. I found strength within myself, not only mentally and spiritually but physically too. I am woman; hear me roar.

I can do all things through Christ which strengtheneth me. (Philippians 4:13)

Toxicity will flow through every vein, ventricle, organ, and crevice like an all-consuming poison. That will slowly eat away at every part of our lives, including our physical health. Sometimes, we are not quite aware that we are slowly being poisoned. We know that something is not right within our lives, but we can't quite put our fingers on the source. We feel fatigued, anxious, and depressed, with low self-esteem and an overall general feeling of being unwell.

Second Corinthians 6:14 tells us that we should not continue with certain relationships:

> Be ye not unequally yoked together with unbelievers: for what fellowship hath righteousness with unrighteousness? and what communion hath light with darkness.

When I read this scripture for the first time, it was puzzling to me, as I felt that it contradicted the second greatest commandment:

> And the second is like unto it, Thou shalt love they neighbour as thyself. (Matthew 22:39)

We are called to love everyone, just as God loved us, but I couldn't understand how to apply this scripture to my life. Even more, why would He call us to love but then not entertain certain relationships?

As I navigated through the toxic relationship, that was part of my problem—I didn't know how to lovingly and rightly apply this scripture while still bringing glory to God. I was filled with shame every time I tried to make it work, only to have it result in another failure. I believed that I wasn't showing enough love; then I thought that Jesus didn't shine through me like He should because if He did, this would work.

This had an avalanche effect on my mental, physical, and spiritual health. After a healthy conversation with my pastor, I realized that I could love from a distance. That is what 2 Corinthians 6:14 allows us to do when there is no other choice for our spiritual health. If we are in a relationship that affects our walk with God, then it is not wise to continue down that path of destruction. Just because we are Christians does not mean we should continue to take abuse in whatever form that takes.

To truly heal yourself daily, you need to train your mind to love from a distance, when needed. You might be disappointed that I don't have a groundbreaking theory to share on how to love from a distance, but perhaps it's better that way. Things that we practice daily, in my opinion, should be kept simple.

Pray for those that hurt you; that is the biggest act of service you could do for anyone. Do you hurt because you yearn to talk with them? When they pop up into your thoughts, pray for them. Pray for whatever battles you know they personally struggle with. Pray that God will work within their hearts and souls, and that they will be healed from their ailments. Do not speak ill of them. It seems easy enough but isn't actually.

When we are hurt, one of our first instincts is to attack the other person verbally and to blame him or her for everything under the sun. Part of our healing is to learn to love that person, despite what he or she has done to us. Then, we must forgive the person, even though that might be hard, especially because, most of the time, the person does not apologize. Why should we forgive someone who has not asked for it? It's for us; it's for our health so that we may walk in an upright manner, knowing that we have given that person the same love that Jesus freely gave us.

As you learn to apply these simple practices in your daily life, you will feel the weight lifted from your shoulders. Play the song "Perfection" by Switch, and remember that, contrary to what you've been told, God sees perfection.

No need to slouch anymore. Learn to love from a distance, and be whole in your healing every day.

1. Who or what in your life is toxic to your health?

2. Identify the effects a toxic relationship has had on you, physically or mentally. (This may take time because you may be unaware of them.)

3. What decision do you need to make for your survival and for your ability to thrive?

4. Ask God to help you heal from this unhealthy relationship. As you begin to heal, pray for the other person, and know it is the best thing you can do. Write down all the things for which you could pray in that person's life.

10

BLOOM

Remember the second-greatest commandment:

> And the second is like unto it, Thou shalt love thy
> neighbour as thyself. (Matthew 22:39)

A popular scripture, for sure, and one we hear preached often,
although it is generally examined from the perspective of loving our
neighbor and what that means for us as Christians. I'd like to focus
on the part that tells us to "love thy neighbor as *thyself*." Have you
ever thought about what that means? What has Jesus asked us to do?
There is a deeper meaning within this scripture, one that is often
missed. He told us to love our neighbors like we love ourselves, but
I'm quite sure He meant to love well and completely.

Hold on, then—that means that we need to love ourselves in
order to have the capacity to love others. Jesus knew how difficult
it would be for us to truly love others if we were unable to love the
beautiful creations that are us. If we do not know what it feels like
to be loved, then it is difficult to emulate the love He gave us.

It can be difficult to love others, partly because we often get hurt
and disappointed, but we are called to love anyway. The idea is that

if we can learn to love ourselves, even with all our shortcomings, flaws, mistakes, and quirks, then we can offer love to others, just as Jesus has done for us.

If we wish to be wholly healed in God, then we cannot ignore this area, even though it is often overlooked, possibly because we also teach that we should not be vain. That is scriptural too, but so is loving ourselves, which means that, again, we need to find balance in our lives. That will allow us to fully embrace who we are in Christ. Loving ourselves is not limited to how we look externally; it is about delighting in what God created us to be.

I certainly understand what it feels like to not love your appearance. As a child, I was often teased about my appearance—from the little hairs on my toes (which apparently wasn't "normal," whatever that means) to my long, skinny "chicken legs" (that's what kids called them), I was a source of laughter. When I told my family about the teasing, my parents would say, "Don't worry; they are just jealous." My mom told me that most girls would kill for long legs like mine. Initially, my response was, "Well, great, they can have them!" They may have been jealous, but what good was that information to me? I just wanted the teasing to stop.

Years later, as I was able to understand what people thought of me, I realized that maybe I disliked who I was on the inside too. I'd hear people describe my characteristics as sensitive, weak, fragile, quiet, and shy. They did not make these statements in a flattering way but with a disquieted tone. It seemed to me that everyone was worried about my personality traits. I learned to dislike these traits, as it felt like they were not something of which I should be proud. These were not things that I learned from someone else; I was made this way by God Himself. For years, though, I hated the way I was built on the inside and felt like I'd never fit in. It was almost a hobby to pick at myself from the inside out and outside in. I believed that I could not do certain things because of my genetic makeup.

The act of self-hate doesn't occur only in kids or teenagers because they are growing into who they are. This can be carried into adulthood, or it even can develop later in life—as adults, we are supposed to be a completed version of ourselves, but occasionally, we don't like the end result. We may have pictured our grown selves a different way, and now we are disappointed with the finished product, but God is never finished with us. We are constantly growing into what He has planned for us. As we go through different seasons, we also grow as they shape who we are.

There was a time when I was at my most vulnerable, and the dislike I had for myself was at its worst. It was a period in my and Jon's life when winter seemed to last all year. Jon is a police officer, a job he dreamed of doing for years. Like any other person who begins within a new organization, he started at the bottom and would work his way up. In law enforcement, that often meant he was assigned to the most isolated and "undesirable" places. There is beauty in everything, but when I say *undesirable*, I'm referring to locations where most people would not choose to live.

We were far up north and away from our family, and everything familiar in our life was a thing of the past. Saying that we had to *adjust* to this type of lifestyle is an understatement; it was culture shock. Jon and I both had a nagging feeling that we didn't fit in. My personality didn't seem to fit in this new adventure. When we were a few months in, I was picking at everything that was wrong with me. Inside and out, I was a mess. Physically, I felt the ramifications from the stress of loathing myself. There were nights when I was physically ill for no apparent reason.

The constant search for a new me was a very present and ever-changing factor while we lived there. I don't know how many times I dyed my hair or cut it, hoping that I would love the "new" me. The change would bring a small dose of confidence for about a week; then I was back where I started. Then there was the war that was going on inside, mainly about my not being good enough because I didn't fit the mold.

When we moved from this posting to our next destination, the stress eased a bit when we relocated closer to home. For years, though,

I continued to struggle with thoughts that were not conducive to accepting who I was made to be. Your physical location doesn't matter if you do not accept yourself. I could have moved a thousand times over and still not loved myself. There likely are exceptions to the rule; some people are extremely good at loving others, even when they don't love themselves. In my experience, though, the capacity I have to love others grows exponentially when I truly love myself. I'm fully aware that I am not perfect, and neither is anyone else, but that doesn't change how much God loves us.

To love who we are is about loving others because when we are capable of fully loving ourselves, we are able to share the love that Jesus has put in us. How can we radiate love when we don't know what it feels like to be loved. When we feel loved, we have a humble confidence that we are enough.

I count myself blessed that my husband wholeheartedly shows his love for me all the time. He truly supports me as a whole, not only about my appearance but about the person I am on the inside.

I remember one instance when I felt absolutely horrible for my mistake. As a maker of headbands, I usually attend a couple of vendor events in any given year. One early fall Saturday morning, the whole family woke early to come with me to this vendor event. We drove forty-five minutes to the event, only to find out that the event was the following Saturday. As I wondered how to break the news, my family looked at me with anticipation, waiting to hear where we could set up. The words finally came out of my mouth, and so did the tears. I said it was all my fault and that I was so very sorry for my mistake. I waited for Jon to be upset or displeased, but he simply looked at me and said, "Oh well. Let's go get some coffee." I was in awe because of his reaction. Why wasn't he angry? We could have been at home, still in pajamas, drinking coffee.

I'm not equating my husband's love to that of God, but it is good imagery. We are also told to love others like God loves us, so it's special when we can see that in others. Jesus will not stop loving us because of our mistakes and shortcomings; rather, He will guide us in the right direction through complete love. We need to ask ourselves if we have genuinely accepted the love that Jesus has offered us. If we saw ourselves as He sees us, love would be so easy for us to receive, and we'd trust that it is real.

> For we are his workmanship, created in Christ Jesus
> unto good works, which God hath before ordained
> that we should walk in them. (Ephesians 2:10)

We are God's masterpiece, created by Him to complete the good things He has planned for us. If we wish to fully complete God's plan for our lives, then we must walk with confidence that we are loved and perfectly made.

My husband, Jon, is a confident guy in most areas of his life. He is humble, yet he knows how to be confident in the tasks he is called to accomplish. I've never pictured him as someone who struggles with the concept of feeling worthy of God's purpose and love. One morning on our deck, while we were enjoying cups of coffee in the fresh summer air, he told me something that knocked me off my chair. He said that the reason he hadn't pursued certain things within the kingdom of God was because he didn't feel worthy of the tasks. He said that he *did* feel loved, but there always has been a part of him that believed he wasn't enough. Other people were more talented or had done this for years, so why would God choose him to do anything important? A part of him had not accepted God's love completely. He didn't even know that about himself, nor was he aware that he was stopping himself from reaching his full potential. Jon felt that he was not worthy of the task, similar to how Moses must have felt when God called him.

To truly be consumed with God's love allows you to walk in His confidence and to consciously accept that you are given the tools to succeed through Him. When you feel that you're enough, you completely live within the love God has for you. Without the element of His unique love, you walk only in your own capacity.

We live in a world where *different* is not exactly a good thing, especially if we are looking for approval from others. The things that make us who we are can either facilitate or inhibit our callings. Jon has the ability to make someone laugh, while making that person feel important at the same time. Those who get to know him realize that the thing they thought was "different" about him is exactly what God called him to be.

Ultimately, the choice is yours. Not a soul on this earth can put your calling into action for you. You can take all your flaws, quirks, and imperfections and turn them into qualities that will work to your advantage. There is nothing wrong with praying for God to help you to be confident with what you believe are flaws and to help you use them for the kingdom, instead of quashing who He's made you to be.

Instead of looking at my sensitive spirit as weakness, what if I viewed it as the ability to be compassionate and show empathy to others? Understanding a person's emotions allows me to be in tune with what they might need in a difficult time in a way that some might miss.

Once we understand that God has made us uniquely and for a purpose, it is much easier to believe we are made just as He intended.

The walk to accepting who you are in Christ can be lonely at times. As you learn to embrace what makes you different, you also might realize that you don't fit in. I believe that as followers of Jesus, we weren't meant to fit in everywhere anyway, so that is a truth you must be willing to accept. Not everyone chooses the path that you have chosen, so it's only natural that you won't be accepted everywhere. I know for sure, though, that to fully accept and love who you are in Christ, you will need to be bold.

Peter and John were told not to speak or teach about the things of Jesus, but they pursued what needed to be done for the kingdom. Even more, it was noticed that there was nothing special about Peter and John. To add injury to insult, they were perceived as unlearned and ignorant. How could these two men speak with such boldness and knowledge, being who they were?

But scripture tells us that the Sanhedrin realized that Peter and

John had been with Jesus. Glory to God! That is what it's all about! Doesn't matter what you think you're capable of. God knows what He can do, through you, to bring Him glory.

> Now when they saw the boldness of Peter and John, and perceived that they were unlearned and ignorant men, they marvelled; and they took knowledge of them, that they had been with Jesus. (Acts 4:13)

Peter and John may not have been considered educated or capable, but they knew who they had been with and who was in them. In knowing this, they did not rely on their own ability but on the all-encompassing Spirit of God.

Being filled with the Spirit of God gives you a supernatural confidence and boldness to which you otherwise would not have access. A popular term for this is *Godfidence*. We can have confidence that God works within us. Therefore, we have the boldness to step out and do things we otherwise wouldn't attempt. He gives us a humbling confidence, and we know that with God by our sides, we can complete His will in our lives.

Only recently I began to pray for God to work within me to a different degree. I prayed that He would use me exactly the way He willed for my life, and I would embrace exactly who I am.

> In the day when I cried thou answeredst me, and strengthenedst me with strength in my soul. (Psalm 138:3)

I prayed that even though I was shy, that He would help me shine His glory.

To allow this to happen, you need to be filled with *Godfidence*. To love yourself is not about high self-esteem or vanity; it's about knowing you are loved by the one who created you. This Godfidence is not about self-love; it's a confidence in knowing that He loves you fully, and you allow yourself to grow in Him. You know that you are worthy of whatever call God decides to put on your life, and according to Him, there is no one better for the job. You are not replaceable or interchangeable. Each and every one of us is unique to God.

During this past year, I have allowed myself to be bolder than ever. At our 2022 youth convention, God spoke to me about my past, telling me that I am not weak, as I believe myself to be, and that I am not my past. This helped me to love myself from His perspective. I've held on to the words and ideals that others have placed on me, when all along, God wanted me to embrace all of myself so that He could use me in the most perfect way. *Perfect* means using all of me according to His will.

I hope that the song "Perfectly Loved" by Rachael Lampa, featuring TobyMac, will speak to your heart today, as you learn that you are perfectly loved. I can guarantee that the ride is not always comfortable, but it is fruitful. When you step out to reveal your true self, including your flaws and insecurities, to others, it often feels foreign and downright wrong. But as you continue to do this, your Godfidence will bloom to new heights.

A plant goes through a season when it doesn't flower. It is only when we, like the plant, go through the winter season, trusting that we are exactly as we are meant to be, that we will bloom.

And who knows what your God-ordained purpose will be as you accept and love yourself the way God does?

1. What do you dislike about yourself? You need to acknowledge how you truly feel before you can love yourself.

2. What have others said about you that you allow to define how you receive and give love?

3. Think about how God could use what you call flaws and insecurities for His greater purpose.

4. In which ways has God been trying to use you, but you feel unworthy of the call?

5. Sit with God for some undisturbed prayer time. Ask Him to use all of you and to help you embrace the real you.

PART III
SOUL

The soul is the very essence of our beings, the only element that is with us eternally. It affects our state of existence here on earth and our future in heaven.

11

MORE THAN ENOUGH

I pray that the following five chapters will provide you with clarity about how essential soul health is. Although all the elements are crucial to your healing, your soul is the cornerstone; it facilitates the function of mind, body, and soul. There is a certain *je ne sais quoi* about soul health; it seems to allow an easier flow of daily healing within the mind and body.

Jesus should be at the center of all aspects of our lives. We could try to achieve mind and body health without His help, but we would not be very successful without Him at the center of these elements. Soul health, though, cannot be achieved without Jesus at the center of it all. It makes sense that if we achieve healing in the depths of our souls, healing mind and body will be that much easier to accomplish.

I hope the next chapters will help to guide you into the healing of your soul through looking at concepts that we often learn to live with.

Let's begin with the concept of being unworthy of love from God and others in your life. When you believe that you are unworthy of His love, anything that He might have for you is unattainable. You might be unaware of the things He has for you because you don't believe any of it is for someone like you. Healing of the soul is a far reach for anyone who believes the lie that "it's just not for people like you." People feel this way for so many reasons. This weapon will pop up time and time again, if not stopped at the get-go.

During my teenage years, I lived through certain events that shook me to my core and changed how I would receive and give love. As I write this, I still feel sickened. My stomach turns, and I want to stop writing. I know, deep down inside, though, that I could help someone by sharing the pain I suffered. That is the thing with pain—no matter how bad it is, it can be a help to someone later. When we are courageous enough to share with others, it will help heal the wound and pain that we may have been hiding for years. It's not only within us but healing for others as it ministers to them.

My parents were always good about letting me stay at a friend's house for sleepovers. My dad dropped me off at my friend's house (I'll call her Anne). What started off as a normal teenage sleepover did not end that way.

Once I got in the house, we did all the things teenage girls do on sleepovers—chatted endlessly, watched a movie, had sleepover snacks that were not at all healthy. Anne then suggested that we sleep outside in the pop-up tent trailer, which sounded like a blast to me.

There are some parts of that night that my mind does not remember, but sometimes I have flashbacks of those moments. Over time, the mind tends to bury certain undesirable memories.

Later that evening, an unexpected male guest arrived. Remember that I was shy, and I wasn't necessarily comfortable with socializing with someone I didn't know. What was I to do? I got over it and tried my best to be sociable. We chatted for what felt like hours in that pop-up trailer. Then Anne thought it would be great to get more snacks. All ready for bed, sitting on the top bunk, I was starting to get tired.

Anne said that it would just take a quick minute, and she'd be right back. I didn't want to be left alone with someone I barely knew, but I thought it would be silly to follow Anne for such a quick trip. As soon the door closed to the camper, the other guest began talking to me. The conversation had a change of tone, but I couldn't quite put my finger on it. I tried to be polite and hold up my end of the conversation as much as I could.

The atmosphere quickly shifted out of nowhere. I was no longer alone on the bunk bed. I found hands on me that shouldn't have been there. I remember feeling stunned and not sure what to do. Unfortunately, no one had told me how to deal with a situation like this because who wants to see this as a reality.

I said, "What are you doing? Get off the bed!" My words had no effect, as the hands that were there before were now trying to fondle me. As I tried to push the hands off, they slid right back just as quickly. Lips kept attempting to kiss me on the lips as I constantly turned my head from left to right. I fought back to the best of my ability, which seemed futile, but I knew that I couldn't stop trying. Everything felt so dirty and revolting. I didn't understand what was going on.

As I was pushed down on the bed, I found my very small body being mounted. I knew at that moment that if I didn't come up with an exit plan quickly, then my life would be changed forever, although it already had. I was a tall but tiny, young girl, without much meat on my bones and even less strength. Arms pinned me down. Eyes attempted to lock with mine, which I tried desperately to avoid. We can look into someone's eyes and feel their emotion; it's an unspoken form of communication. If I could help it, there was no way I would allow anyone to have access to something so profound.

Then I found some sort of super-girl strength within me. I pushed up with my arms and turned the lower part of my body as hard as I could. What happened next was glorious; I know that God was there with me that night. He flew off the bed—the top bunk—and plummeted to the floor. I heard a hard thump and quickly looked down to see if he was injured. His fury was both satisfying and terrifying at the same time. Of course, I had no doubt that I had done the right thing. When Anne came back, suddenly the room's atmosphere became quiet and still. I realized that he had no intention of letting on about what had happened. I felt so dirty and alone. All I could think was that nobody would believe me. *I'm nothing, and who am I to cause trouble over something that is perhaps normal?* As a teenager, I had no idea what was acceptable. It felt wrong, but maybe I was overreacting.

I now know that this is a common mistake made by those who are sexually assaulted—they believe that they are at fault. *You're being too sensitive*, they think. *Get over it; no one really cares.*

When I went home the next day, didn't think about it too much. In fact, I had quickly buried it deep within me. This was shameful and should never be spoken about, not even to my parents. What had I done that had made him believe he could touch me that way? Again, I blamed myself for that horrible act that was out of my control. I had not asked for that. All I had done was be sociable in the most normal way.

Looking back on this, I wish I had told my parents. They could have helped me. It would have helped me to talk about it and to hear from them that it was not my fault. Children are helpless and innocent. This is part of the reason that I ask my children a million questions, and I do not like sleepovers, especially at the house of a friend we have not met or that we don't know very well. As parents, it is our job to protect our children, including from things of which they are unaware.

Later in high school, there was another situation that was difficult for me—my parents' divorce. Isn't divorce difficult for all children? Unfortunately, it was the type of divorce when everything went sideways. Hearts were broken and filled with disappointment and the feeling that life would never be normal. My dad needed to start fresh after everything was finished. He was a born-and-raised Quebecer and still had lots of family within Quebec. Naturally, that was the location where he asked to be transferred. As I was already living with him, it just seemed right for me to follow.

I was a teenager, a time in my life when I was discovering who I was going to be, what was important to me, and who I wanted to become. Change can be good, although most of the time, we do not enjoy the transition. Attending a new school meant that I would have to find my place among groups of friends who already had formed. I felt like I didn't know myself, much less where I belonged.

Teenagers naturally struggle with finding who they are; it is part of the process. Strong adult figures in a teenager's life aids them in navigating through the confusion of growing up. Support from people they can trust and lean on is an integral part of their making smart decisions.

As I continued to get to know the various groups within my school, I developed a circle of friends. But then, something happened, and I began hanging out with the wrong crowd. Looking back, it's clear to me now that the entire group felt unworthy and simply not enough. I personally felt that was where I belonged. Who was I to aim for more? My past haunted the decisions I continued to make as a teenager. My dad, bless his heart, never asked too many questions. As long as I seemed happy and healthy, then surely everything was good. He did enforce a curfew and told me not to do drugs or drink alcohol, but I had become stealthy, enabling me to hide the drug and alcohol use—or so I believed. Maybe he did know about my transgressions, but because of the way he was raised, he let them slide. He was from a generation in which drinking, drugs, and everything in between was part of the growing-up process.

Unworthy, unloved, and rejected people make very bad decisions. Why? They will do whatever it takes to be loved, even if that means doing things that make them feel more unworthy in the attempt to be worthy. It's a vicious cycle that's seen mostly by loved ones, looking in from the outside.

Most of the time, I didn't think about how I felt. My search for the next validation went into overdrive. Everything was blurry, my brain was in a fog, and I simply *did*. Combine my past experience of sexual assault with my parents' divorce and a new school for me, and it was a recipe for disaster.

Some of my new habits were not coming home almost all weekend and partying with alcohol and marijuana. I had a curfew so it was so much simpler to just sleep over at my friend's house. Everything felt so dark at that time. Without knowing it, I had shut the door to the rest of the world. I was quite happy with falling off the grid and continuing down this path of destruction. The boys I chose to date were less than desirable. I always chose someone with no ambition, no moral values, and no care for a thing in the world. That was because I was convinced I deserved to be with someone like that. Who would want me anyway? I would be lucky to get a guy to give me the time of day.

In all of this, another life changing event happened from time to time. I've blocked out most of those memories for self-preservation purposes, but I remember being touched, caressed, and violated, this time in a small basement room—the brush of a hand against my neck that slowly moved across my body. In between all this, he would play his computer games, while I felt frozen. This whole situation felt so confusing. I felt like a toy that he played with.

The reoccurring thought that haunts me is that I couldn't move. This time the assault was gentle and calculated, which perhaps was worse than the first experience, as it felt like I was slowly being deceived. My mind played tricks on me because it occurred in this manner. *It's only a little gentle touching. What is wrong with that?* There was no aggressive behavior, but my space was violated nonetheless, and I felt so dirty and powerless. I couldn't just throw this one off the bunk bed. How could I defend my someone who was being "gentle"?

As I share this with you, tears well up in my eyes. How could I have let this happen? Why didn't I fight back or say something? *Unworthy.* Unworthy of better, of love, and of respect.

A story in the New Testament speaks about the faith of a centurion. In Matthew 8, we read that the centurion had a servant at home who was paralyzed. This centurion came to Jesus, asking Him to heal his servant who was tormented by this illness. Jesus quickly said that He would go and heal him, meaning that He wanted to enter the centurion's home. But just as quickly as Jesus said that, the centurion expressed that he was not worthy of Jesus entering his home. He suggested that Jesus could just speak and heal his servant from where they were.

Matthew 8:8 shows the unworthiness that the centurion felt:

> The centurion answered and said, Lord, I am not worthy that thou shouldest come under my roof; but speak the word only, and my servant shall be healed.

Jesus was wowed that day by the faith this man held within him. The centurion believed in Jesus so much that he knew that all that was required of Jesus was to speak the word. I'd like to point out, though, that the centurion felt that he was not worthy to have Jesus in his home. He was acutely aware of the power Jesus held but had categorized himself as unworthy.

How often do you know what Jesus can do for you, but you block Him out because of your unworthiness? You don't see yourself as enough to invite Him into your home. Perhaps someone has spoken to you about the love Jesus has for you, but you conclude that it is not for people like you. The person speaking into your life cannot possibly know all the things you've done or lived through. The stain from your past is too deep and has been sitting far too long; it is past the point of redemption. No one could possibly understand how you're feeling, much less love you. You live vicariously through others as you watch Jesus work in their lives. You have carried the shame and unworthiness for so long that you no longer feel it weighing you down. You don't hear the knock of Jesus at your door because you don't believe it is possible.

No matter from where our unworthiness stems, the shame we

carry stops us from pursuing our whole healing in God. The feeling of unworthiness runs deep when we carry it around with us. When we don't believe there is any other way to live, then we simply continue living beneath what Jesus has planned for us.

This is exactly what I did throughout my teenage years and well into adulthood. I believed that I was not worth the time and effort. There is a song called "The Father's House" by Cory Asbury that speaks directly to this. The lyrics say, "Failure won't define me; that's what my Father does." This is what I hope you will carry with you in your heart as you listen to the song. You need to let Jesus define you. There is room in *your* Father's house for you. Bring your unworthiness, and let Him make something beautiful with it.

One Saturday morning, as I was rushing home after a night of partying, I had to make a pit stop behind a random apartment building because I didn't want to vomit on the side of the road. I felt just wretched; I had consumed too much alcohol.

As I walked in the door, I saw that my father had already started his day and was in full cleaning mode. This time, he did notice that I was not looking especially vibrant, and he asked if I was all right. To my surprise, he accepted my simple answer—I had gone to bed really late and was tired. I headed downstairs to clean myself up and get some sleep.

School was always somewhat easy for me, except for math, where the struggles I had were out of this world. (I still do not like it and sometimes use my fingers to calculate math answers.) The Lord blesses us all differently, and He apparently didn't think I needed math skills. I really loved the language classes, but I used to fall asleep in my English class, which seemed odd to me because I enjoyed English overall. Even with my brief naps, I still did well, considering the lack of attention I seemed to have. However, deep down I knew my grades could be far better . I wasn't failing but they weren't stellar. I didn't practice study habits during this time when darkness was taking over all areas of my life. God knew me, but I didn't know Him. My mom had spoken to us about Jesus in the past, but that didn't mean anything because I didn't have a relationship with Him.

That summer, my dad found a job for me that was a teenaged girl's dream—an overnight babysitting job that paid more money than I knew what to do with. All I had to do was show up for bedtime and then watch movies while the kids slept or until I fell asleep myself. Then, at around six o'clock in the morning, I was off the hook and went home. I was able to work this job during the week because it was essentially a well-paid sleepover.

As money started to roll in, I saw how real life worked. A friend of mine was experiencing a very difficult time in her life. Her family did not have much money for groceries after covering other expenses. This broke my heart. I had always been fortunate enough to never experience missing a meal, and I couldn't imagine how hard that must be. So I would go to the corner store and buy canned goods, Kraft dinners, Pop-Tarts, or anything that could be appropriate for a "meal." I believe that this was the beginning of the end of my dark era. I felt a sense of purpose as I walked to the store, and love filled my heart on my trek to drop off the groceries off with my friend's family.

Perhaps the best way to see light in your own life is to be the light in the life of others. Although it would be years before I completely gave my life to God, there is no doubt that He had already started working. I was battling with unworthiness, feeling I wasn't enough, and feeling unloved, and this had hung on to me for far too long. As I grew up, I was forced to see the future. Helping a friend with real-world problems opened my eyes.

Of the many relationships I had in this period of my life, two stick out like sore thumbs. I was so sure my papa would be pleased with the first one. Unfortunately my dad was unable to understand what was being said. No joke, there was no articulation in his speech whatsoever. My dad tried hard to strike up a conversation with this dude, but every answer left him more confused. Needless to say, this relationship never took off.

Then I thought I'd found a relationship that was worth the risk. Unfortunately, that relationship lasted only a short time, as I was on the receiving end of physically aggressive behavior. I felt as if being my own separate person was not an option, and everything required his approval. One day, we began to argue again—I can't remember what the issue was—but all of a sudden, he was shaking me. Instead of being in shock or confused, I ended things on the spot. This was impressive, as months before that, I likely would have taken the abuse and not fought back. Of course, he gave gifts and apologies, but that incident was my *enough*!

One person tried to convince me that I should give him another chance. "People make mistakes," the person said. Seriously? I know the person thought that my former partner was being kind in trying to make amends. I never said that I hadn't forgiven him. I had just decided that I'd had enough. How many mistakes by the people around me would I be subject to before I could think about my well-being?

At about the same time, something clicked in my mind. I don't know which event led to this wake-up call, but the crucial part is that it happened. Between the poor grades, bad boyfriends, late-night partying, and more bad decisions, I decided that I needed to try to be better. The way in which I was living did not coincide with my hopes and dreams. I was in my senior year of high school, so it was now or never. I at least had to try. Weekend parties became a thing of the past, and late-night study sessions became the new norm. My friends were not impressed with this sudden change, and we had many hard conversations. It wasn't about them; this was about my future and my dreams.

Remember that there always will be at least one person who does not agree with a change in your life. You need to hold on to your *why* even more in these instances. Your mind will attack you, and unworthiness will creep back into your life.

This book has been a long time coming, but I cannot tell you how many times I have thought, *Who am I to write this book? There are so many other books written by worthy authors.* But who's to say

I am not worthy of writing a book? This is my story, given to me by God Himself, and there isn't a soul on earth who can take that away from me.

To feel unworthy is to live through much darkness and pain. Most times, it feels like there is no light in your life.

> This is the message we have heard from Him and
> announce to you, that God is Light, and in Him
> there is no darkness at all. (1 John 1:5)

God is light, so when you feel unworthy and as if there is no light in your life, it would be normal to wonder where He is within it. To turn on the light is to allow Him to work in your life.

When we were expecting our fourth child, Jon and I were both awakened from a dead sleep by a bright light. The ceiling fan in our room has a light, and we had put the remote that controls the light between our pillows. One of us must have rolled over and hit the right button, as out of nowhere, our room went from complete darkness to blinding light. I jumped to a sitting position, clasping my extremely pregnant belly, with frightened breathing, wondering who was attacking us. Jon was startled by my reaction, and it took a minute for us to realize what was going on.

God is like that. You can feel surrounded by complete darkness one minute, but when He decides to show up and light up your world, watch out!

Do not be misled into believing that He is not there when life gets dark. We have the power to press that button and cast out darkness in His name. Psalm 139:7–8 tells us that God is everywhere; He is omnipresent:

> Where can I go from your Spirit? Where can I flee
> from your presence? If I go up to the heavens, you
> are there; if I make my bed in the depths, you are
> there.

Whether or not you choose to acknowledge God's presence is up to you, but He is there. If you do not call out to Him, lean on Him, and put all your trust in Him, it can be difficult to feel His presence. Jesus will only enter a place into which He's been invited. Did you forget to send the invitation? All the chaos that surrounds you may cause you to forget who needs to be called on—that's the point of chaos that comes from the enemy.

We get so caught up in our circumstances and emotions, that our souls forget who the great I AM is. We must stop looking at our problems and start searching for the solution. We are not unworthy because of the darkness we have seen and experienced.

Many modern lighting systems include a dimmer so you can choose how bright the light shines in that room. To go from darkness to light, you slowly turn the switch until it reaches your desired brightness. Your relationship with Jesus is just like that dimmer. *You* choose how much of Him to let in. You have the power to allow His presence to flood the whole room. Every person chosen in the Bible was flawed and had sinned. Many of them felt the depths of darkness. I dare say that made them more qualified to shine God's light. The darkness you have seen has been preparing you for your purpose. Because you have seen and felt darkness, you know the power and depth of His light. Your testimony is greater because of the test.

Do you feel unworthy of the love Jesus wants to instill in you? Good news—we are all unworthy of His love. Not one soul on earth is worthy. Perhaps that's the "secret message" that we need to shout from the rooftop. It is why Jesus had to come down from heaven and die on the cross—so that we could have salvation through Him. He does not want us to hold on to being unworthy; it's that even with all our sins and flaws, He still loves us. The love that parents have for their children is similar to this concept. Children are constantly taught what to do and not do. Nearly every day, they are reprimanded for some action or something they said wrong. As a parent, I can tell you that my love never fades for my children, even when I have to discipline them.

On the day I wrote this chapter, I spoke with my tribe about responsibilities and time management as I was preparing their peanut butter sandwiches for school. I firmly believe that if you do not give children certain tasks, they will be hindered later in life. In our home, our children fold their own clothes, clean the cat litter, take out the garbage, and clean their play area, to name a few chores. There are times when they give me the stink eye for enforcing these tasks, but I know it is for their good. If I don't show them how to be responsible and manage their time, who will? Later in life, as they become adults, it will be much more difficult to learn these lessons in addition to everything else life will throw at them.

Continuing my very long speech that morning, I said, "I know you guys think I'm horrible because of these rules."

Then my ten-year-old, seeming in shock and close to anger, said, "We do *not* think you're horrible! How dare you even think that?"

It caught me off guard; even after I'd told them that if the chores weren't done, they would lose screen time, my son did not dislike me. This was similar to when God is teaching me something; it might be frustrating, but I never think that He is horrible. I know that He is guiding me to be who I was meant to be. There is no need to feel unworthy because of this.

When I discipline my children, I never believe they are not worthy of my love or that they are a lost cause. In fact, it drives me to show them love even more because I want them to know that when *Maman* is angry, she still loves them. God's love is like that. Stop believing the lies in your head. Jesus does not love you less because of your past mistakes and sins.

One of the most common reasons that people don't attend church is that they feel unworthy or that they don't belong. Perhaps you feel you're not perfect enough, or you've made too many mistakes. Maybe it's something you've gone through that was not your fault. I've said it previously, and I will say it again: no one is worthy, but God loves you. He wants you to turn toward Him that much more, allowing His love to cover your past. Stop carrying the burden of your sins. You will never be able to heal while carrying that weight.

God wants to take that heavy weight from you. Whether you carry a ten-pound or ninety-five-pound dumbbell, it's all the same to Him. Jesus died at Calvary for *you* and your sins! Don't waste the grandest gesture of love this world has ever seen. Allow His light to shine within you. Allow Jesus's love to make you whole and complete as He heals you. Remember that you cannot receive that of which you do not believe you are worthy.

1. What past or present experiences do you carry with you? Write them down, along with how they make you feel.

2. Are these experiences blocking you from receiving your healing and all that God has for you?

3. Would someone in your life benefit from you shining the love of Jesus in his or her life? What could you do to show that love?

4. We are all unworthy but saved by grace. How does this change your perspective going forward?

5. Are you ready to believe you're enough and to receive God's full healing and purpose within your life? Write down one way you can take a step toward claiming that.

12

HIDING FAWN

We are all dealt a different hand in life. The events that are put in our lives are meant to shape us and for us to minister to others as we come out on the other side. We do not go through the same things, and our reactions are not identical either. Sure, some events resemble another person's experience, but there are slight differences within those situations. I believe that God does this for a reason; through the differences, we can help others.

There is always a greater purpose when you go through a struggle. Because you experienced it differently, you have a different perspective. This is similar to the concept of looking in from the outside.

The lot I've been handed in life is to walk through certain experiences alone. I do not proclaim this for pity but to share with you a very important part of healing in Christ. Unquestionably, it has been difficult to see others surrounded by friends and family who offer them support. Within my struggles, though, a part of me has wished to have the support with which others seem blessed. When I feel alone, my heart aches for companionship. I've been blessed with four beautiful children and a loving husband, and my heart has been filled with thanksgiving that depends on my little tribe.

Often, we hear the message that we are not meant to be alone, that we require each other's fellowship for a healthy state of mind, and that God did not create us to do this life alone. Scripturally, this is true, God created woman so that man would have a companion; it was not good for him to be alone. The flip side, however, seems to be just as important. Learning to be alone with God is part of our healing process and plays a crucial role for us to be whole in Him. It requires us to give our whole heart and trust to Him.

As a mom of four, my finding time to be alone can be quite challenging. Another human being constantly is following me and requiring something from me. Furthermore, being a mom of a toddler makes it more difficult to find time alone—even going to the bathroom. Just this morning, as I was about to jump in the shower, this little person followed me into the bathroom, even though I had just told her that she was to hang out with her big sister while I got ready for the day. But she wanted to be with me, even if that meant lying on the bathroom floor while she waited. She will lie on the floor as I take a shower, playing with little her pal "Didiche," which is a pink stuffed sloth. It doesn't bother me to have her there, but it seems I'm never alone. I can't remember a time when I've gone on vacation to be by myself. Normally, I'm traveling to meet someone or going somewhere with the whole family. Jon and I love to spend time with one another, so even when we were dating, we'd do all things together.

This past year, the Lord has required some big steps on my part in my healing process. I'm thankful that He has done it ever so gently. Over the course of a few months, He's walked with me with a spiritual healing in mind. Since I don't have much experience in being alone, this was a foreign and scary concept for me. I do not know how to be alone. The idea of going somewhere without a friend or my family causes me anxiety. *What will I do, alone? What if something horrible happens, and nobody is there to help me? What if something happens to my family while I'm gone? I need to stick around so I can make sure everyone is OK.* This scenario screams too much control on my part and a lack of trust in God!

When you are unaccustomed to being alone, you depend on others around you in all areas of your life. As I've said many times, I have a good husband who would do anything for me and our family. I have become very dependent on the sense of security he provides, just by being who he is. This may sound so lovely, romantic, and what every person hopes for in a relationship—or maybe you wonder if I'm my own person. I am very much an independent woman with her own thoughts and dreams. Jon can attest that I speak my mind, perhaps too much sometimes. I am known to have a stubborn side. In fact, you can find me building furniture, painting, mowing the lawn, and using the barbecue, but I still love having my other half to rely on.

I've experienced doing life without Jon by my side. When he was away for six months of intensive training, I was home alone with our toddler, while pregnant with our now-twelve-year-old daughter. I gave birth to her without Jon at my side—now, that was a trying time. I have a strong relationship with Jon. We are there for each other through thick and thin. But we—all of us—can reach a level of dependency on those around us where we no longer rely on God for our strength.

This isn't limited to people; it also includes things and habits that we form in our lives for comfort. We grow dependent on those items or habits so that they become the comfort and strength in our lives. Maybe it's a certain routine that we've implemented in our lives, and without it, we would not know how to cope. Routine is good in life; it's healthy, but when we need something to happen at a certain time, or we need a specific item to function, that is dependency. We need to ask ourselves, *Am I placing more trust in my routine than I put in God?*

Because of the pandemic, I am guilty of this, 100 percent. I had built such a solid daily routine from morning to evening that when things started to change, I was startled, not only mentally but spiritually. My soul was shaken to a point that I didn't know what to do with myself. Life was getting back to normal, which is what I wanted, so why did I feel so out of place?

As my spiritual life deepened, things within my soul and mind seemed to be shaken even more. I enjoy waking up to see a sunrise and to spend alone time with God, especially before my tribe awakes for the day. This sacred time with God was part of the core foundation of my healing in Him, but it was often disturbed by a restless night's sleep or no sleep at all. Waking up in a panic and then attempting to go back to sleep became a part of my life. It was difficult to stay on course with early mornings when I was bothered in such a way. I knew deep down, though, that somehow, I'd have to push through, that this was part of the whole. There is something healing in being alone with God. Even with all the time in the morning that I was giving Him, this was not the whole healing I was required to learn. He wanted more of me. I just didn't quite understand where He was taking me yet.

This year, my grandpa became quite ill. Because I'm so close with my grandparents, we decided I should go for a visit. This part of my family lives in the beautiful province of British Columbia, perhaps one of my favorite places on earth. Again, because of the pandemic, I hadn't seen them for years. I went alone—no kids at all, not even my youngest, Esmée, from whom I had not been apart since her birth. Internally, I was at war with two different emotions: excitement about going on vacation alone, and fear of not having my support system with me. I knew, though, that if I didn't go then, I would regret not jumping at the opportunity to visit with my grandpa.

As I arrived at my destination, I could hear the pitter-patter sound of the rain hitting the ground at the Victoria, British Columbia, airport. Clouds were sweeping across the sky, and I could tell that the sun would not make an appearance that day. I felt nostalgic as memories flooded my mind and heart from my childhood. The excitement I felt from the hustle and bustle at the airport arrivals was contagious, as people greeted each other with great joy and exhilaration. I imagined a grandmother meeting her grandson for the first time, a family hugging and jumping on each other after a long time apart. I had never been in this airport when it was so busy. Travelers waited patiently for their bags to arrive on the conveyor belt. There was an atmosphere of love, and everywhere I looked, someone was smiling from ear to ear.

In British Columbia, rain is a regular occurrence. It's as normal as a twenty-degrees-below-zero January day in Canada's capital. Perhaps because it had been so long since I'd visited, I found the rain soothing and somehow poetic. My luggage came quickly, and I felt ready for a week of "me time," something I hadn't experienced in nearly three years.

I easily found a bench and sat down as I waited for my ride to arrive and for my journey to begin. I was excited as I looked at every entrance with anticipation. Approximately twenty minutes went by, and I thought it might be wise to call my ride. *No, no,* I told myself, *just be patient. Wait at least another ten minutes.* The time went by quickly, and I decided it was time to check on my ride.

When I called, my ride picked up on the other end—and my heart dropped a little. Unfortunately, there was a miscommunication, and the days were mixed up. My ride was nowhere near the airport. We eventually decided that I should take a cab to the ferry; that was the best decision in that particular situation.

Victoria is not like any other city; the entire province of British Columbia is hard to compare to other Canadian provinces. It's like a little world in itself between the ocean and humongous trees. To get where I was going was not just a simple car ride. I needed to cross the ocean—hence, the reason for the ferry ride (one of my fondest childhood memories). I could jump on the ferry as a foot passenger and reach my destination in half the time it would have taken my ride to get to the airport.

Still, regardless of the reason for the mishap, my heart was hurt. I felt forgotten and alone, and that is not enjoyable. People do not forget things on purpose; in fact, if you ponder the definition of forget, you'll realize that it's an accident. Nobody forgets to eat on purpose, but it happens; I'm sure I'm not the only one who gets busy and forgets to eat. When we feel light-headed, faint, and maybe a little nauseated, then we realize that we haven't eaten anything. Car accidents happen, yet just because they are accidents doesn't ease the pain of the injuries incurred.

I cried on my little bench in the airport while trying to pull myself together. I felt alone and wondered why this was happening. At times, tears get us through to the next step, although this is not to be mistaken for weakness. Hiding our emotions is where we can go wrong. I called Jon, and he helped me get together. He told me that he was praying for me. I sat there for another five minutes; then I picked myself up and headed out the airport doors.

The rain had gone from feeling comforting to depressing as my mind slowly started to switch. As mentioned, the mind is a powerful thing, and we must gird it at all times. With very little experience in grabbing a cab, I selected the first one waiting at the exit doors of the airport. The cab driver hopped out of the cab with a chipper attitude and grabbed my bags with so much joy. I thought, *Wow, he is joyful. This is odd.* I'd probably seen too many movies in which cab drivers are quiet and even grumpy, so I thought all of them were that way. Still, they had a right to be grumpy after driving others around all day, and not all customers are grateful or polite.

As I settled in my seat, I grabbed my phone, thinking this would be a quiet cab ride. The driver asked where I was headed and where home was for me.

At that point, I thought, *Dude, I don't really want to chat. Just let me wallow.*

He was insistent, though. We conversed about the rain in Victoria and the cold in Ottawa. If I had been standing, what happened next would have knocked me off my feet—he began to talk about God. I believe that a large percentage of the population would rather not speak about God; it can even be seen as a taboo subject. This cab driver, however, didn't just mention God; he went on and on about God's goodness.

"People are never happy," he said. "It's never enough, and they always need more. One day, we are unhappy because it's raining or snowing; the next day, we complain about the heat. We need to realize that God is enough, and we have all we could ever need in Him."

This man was delighting in the goodness of God right in front of me. I knew right then that God was showing me that I was not forgotten or alone. *Blessed* doesn't begin to describe how I felt in that moment. This experience was surreal. *Who am I*, I wondered, *that God would make a point to remind me of what I mean to Him?*

When we feel forgotten, we then often feel unloved, not valuable, and unimportant, but scripture tells us otherwise:

> But even the very hairs of your head are all numbered. Fear not therefore: ye are of more value than many sparrows. (Luke 12:7)

> Before I formed you in the womb I knew you; Before you were born I sanctified you; I ordained you a prophet to the nations. (Jeremiah 1:5)

How can a God who knows the number of hairs on your head, a God who knew you before you were formed, forget you or leave you alone?

Little did I know that this was the beginning of another step in my journey to healing me as a whole. God was slowly teaching me how to be comfortable with being alone with Him, which is now so very clear to me as a need in our healing in the soul.

While I was on Salt Spring Island, visiting my grandparents, many instances of God's presence were apparent to me. The punches kept coming at me, and it was hard to comprehend why I was going through this. At the same time, I could feel His constant and unfailing love as I walked through unknown territory. One moment in particular stuck with me, and I doubt I'll ever shake the palpable love I felt that day.

As a child I would play and dream in my grandparents' backyard, which is more like an enchanted forest—acres and acres of huge green trees, all surrounded by lustrous wild vegetation. A tiny babbling brook flows through the entrance of the forest, where I always saw frogs and lily pads. When I was encircled by the trees that were larger than life, I couldn't help but feel the majesty of the one who created it all.

As I stepped out for some air on that rainy morning, my soul needed respite from all that had gone on. Step after step, I climbed the little hill up through the trees, and moss and sticks crunched under my feet. I came to a stop for just a moment to embrace the beauty of all that surrounded me. One minute before that, the clouds had darkened the sky. But as I looked up through the tall branches of the trees, which almost seemed to touch the sky, the sun broke through and shimmering rays fell on me. I thought that the gratitude I felt in that moment was all I needed.

Turning around to soak it all in, I saw a fawn staring at me. Nestled among the green vegetation, it stood still about ten steps away, looking into my eyes. At first, I thought the fawn would quickly scurry away, but it just stood there. We looked at each other for a long time, and I felt the presence of God so strongly. As I began to praise and worship right there, tears rolled down my face. It was yet another instance in which the Lord showed me that I was not alone. I simply had to find Him in the secret places. Basking in this moment, I stood there for a long time, not wanting to let this piece of time fade away.

Did you know that a mother deer will choose a hiding place for her fawn? She does that to protect their baby, as her presence may attract predators. She always comes back to nurse her fawn and never has a problem finding it, as the chosen place is isolated but known to her. If, for some reason, the fawn leaves this hiding place, it is trained to go back to the last place its mother left it. I researched this because I was so taken by my experience with the fawn.

As I continued to read about a fawns' behavior, I wondered how God does the same with us. Although God is everywhere all the time, there is a secret place where we can find Him. It's the place we go to feed our souls. Only we and God know about this place. Not only can we find Him in this place, but we should always return to it for this time of solitude with Him.

Have you ever read something and known that it was for you, as if God knew that you needed it? This happened for me as I was reading *The Book on Prayer* by Ken Gurley, in which he speaks about a "trysting place." A trysting place is a location where lovers meet at a set time. In Exodus 32–33, we read about Moses building a tabernacle outside of the camp or far from the rest of the community. This was to be a place where everyone could go to meet with the Lord. Before this happened, the people worshipped idols, followed by Moses pleading with God not to destroy them because of their great sin.

After Moses pitched this tabernacle, he would go inside alone. A cloudy pillar would come down and stand at the door, and then he would talk with God. The people saw this cloudy pillar, which prompted them to worship God in all His glory. Moses spoke to God as friends would speak with each other. This place was isolated from the rest of community; it was a meeting place where Moses and others could speak to and worship God.

I believe two concepts are important within those chapters. The first is that the meeting place needed to be far from the distractions of everyday life; it was a sacred and quiet place. The second is that this was what the people needed spiritually, a place where they could have one-on-one time with God. They needed to have access to Him personally.

It is a privilege that we have full access to God whenever we want. We do not need to ask a priest or pastor to speak with Him on our behalf. We need a "trysting place" where only we and God meet, outside of the hustle and bustle of everyday life.

Upon my return from British Columbia, the Lord continued to slowly work on me with regard to being alone. Deep down, I knew my inability to be alone was a problem. I had a dependency on others instead of on Jesus. I yearned to have alone time, but on the other hand, I was filled with fear at the idea.

As I continued to write this book in the following months, I thought how great it would be to get away for a few days, solely for purpose of fully concentrating on the writing process. Surprisingly, an opportunity and blessing were placed in my hands to go away for four days all by myself. At first, I jumped at the idea. Jon and I made all the plans required (necessary when there are kids at home). As departure day approached, however, I was filled with fear again and believed this was a horrible idea. Have you ever known that something was good for you but you refused to do it? That was the predicament I was battling. I knew that this was an excellent opportunity, but I didn't have the guts to do it. I tried to find reasons for why I shouldn't go—mainly, it was that my kids needed me to care for them.

Regardless of the fact that Jon had it handled, and my fifteen-year-old son, Liam, was game to help out, I needed confirmation that this was what God wanted for me and that He would be with me. So I went to Him in prayer, asking for the only opinion that really mattered. The answer didn't surprise me that much. God impressed on my heart that this was exactly what He required of me and that I was to learn to be alone with Him.

Even more, this was part of the healing process because the problem was that I still was holding something back. Full trust in Him from within me was not whole. The reason I didn't want to be alone was that I still relied on others too much. The trust I had in others outweighed the trust I had in God at times. But as I embarked on this four-day journey, it was well and evident in my soul that this was the path God wanted me to walk.

The days I spent alone were far better than I expected them to be, and I experienced the beauty of quiet and stillness with God.

I knew that He was enough and learned how to place all my trust in Him.

Why is learning to be alone part of the soul-healing process? As you take the time to create a trysting place, you will see it carried into your everyday life. You will learn that God is omnipresent and within you, and that secret place becomes Him in you. You will fully rely on Him as a whole. You will learn that as you walk this life, sometimes alone, you really aren't alone when you make a trysting place within you.

My twelve-year-old daughter, Novalee, was in tears, and her heart ached this week because she felt like she did not fit in anywhere. She watched other friends bond and spend special time together, and she wondered why she wasn't invited. We sat together and talked about how she felt, but then she wanted to go to her room. Novalee was still crying, so I said to her, "Don't go to your room. You'll be alone."

As quickly as the words had come from mouth, she said, "I'm not alone. I have Jesus."

Liam laughed and exclaimed in teenager lingo, "Oh Maman, you got wrecked!"

I was so proud of my girl that even in her pain, she knew who held her.

Daily healing in our souls is found in the secret place. As a fawn is trained to return to its hiding place, we also need that innate response as we do everyday life. The hiding place is for our protection, just as the deer hides its baby. God can be that secret place—a place where He will cover, protect, heal, and guide us as we learn to carry the hiding place with us everywhere.

Know that you are never alone and that He is simply a whisper away. The fawn may feel alone at times, but the mom always knows where her baby is. The God who created you knows where you are and what you need. Come to Him and claim your healing as you hide under His wings.

He shall cover thee with His feathers, And under
His wings you shall take refuge; His truth shall be
your shield and buckler. (Psalm 91:4)

Play the song "The Secret Place" by Phil Wickham. I pray that
you are brave enough to find that trysting place—the place where
you may find rest, peace, and certainly healing through it all.

1. Can you identify someone or something that you might be relying on instead of God?

2. What habits have you formed that keep you from the trysting place?

3. Look back and find three times when God showed up in an unexpected way when you felt very alone. It is good practice to reminisce and thank God for what He's already done.

4. What place in your home or life can you predetermine as a place to meet with God on a daily basis?

5. Now that you have chosen a place, play the song "The Secret Place" by Phil Wickham and begin to commune with God as you would with a friend.

13

JOY IS A CHOICE

One of the most important steps to the daily healing of our souls is to be filled with God's joy. I'd like to clarify that this is not the same emotion we call happiness or the joy that this world so loudly speaks of. This is an eternal joy, one that is not dependent on our situation. It's not reliant on anything else in this life; it's purely based on the relationship we have with Jesus. It's a joy that can only be harvested through an entirely dependent heart in Jesus. Through loss and grief, I have learned that the only sustainable joy we could ever hope for is that which is found in Jesus.

Loss is described as "the fact or process of losing something or someone" or "the state or feeling of grief when deprived of someone or something of value." You can lose joy in your life through the circumstances you go through. Or perhaps you never had God's joy, and that is what you desperately need. I've often heard that someone lost so-and-so and has never been the same. This sentiment is true when you lose something significant in your life. You are changed, whether or not you have come to terms with it. As an individual, you have the power to decide how circumstances change you. The question remains: how will you allow it to shape the present and future you?

I will never forget the feeling of losing my babies. My husband and I now have four wonderful blessings, but I suffered through two miscarriages. I technically did not miscarry because both times, my body did not do its job to miscarry. I had to undergo a dilation and curettage procedure (D&C), which was almost harder for me to come to terms with.

The first time, I rushed to the hospital because there was bleeding in what seemed like a normal pregnancy. We had just moved from our northern posting and felt ready to add to our family of three.

On that fall evening, our children were fast asleep for the night. I was enjoying some downtime, watching my favorite show, *Gilmore Girls*.

Once the kids were in bed, it was a sacred time for me. I could sit back, relax, decompress, and be me before starting it all the next day. Jon was on a night shift. Back then, it was normal for us; I was used to chilling alone.

But on that rainy evening, my world was turned upside down. All of a sudden, I felt that something was not right. I rushed to the bathroom, as I suspected there was bleeding. I immediately fell to the floor and started to cry and panic. Something was wrong; I just knew it. I tried to control my panicked breathing and picked up the phone to call Jon. Thank God, he was able to answer right away—in his line of work, that was not always possible. I told him what had happened but I wasn't doing very well in keeping my composure.

"I'm coming home," he said. The plan was that he would come home, and I'd go to the hospital.

As I waited for him to arrive, I called my ol' bean— we all need someone to talk to in a crisis. As usual, she talked with me and helped me stay calm, but her most important action was to pray with me. We prayed on the phone that night for God to have His hand on my baby and me. We prayed that He would comfort and strengthen me as I waited for an answer from the doctor.

Peace always covers me when I enter into prayer. I don't believe

I have ever prayed and been anxious at the same time. The anxiety and stress may come back afterward, but in prayer, there is an indescribable peace. When I focus on God and allow His presence to work in my situation, nothing in this world can compare to it.

Of course, my friend was so positive, repeating over and over that everything was surely fine. I needed someone to be positive for me because my mind was quickly going down the rabbit hole. Don't we do this in a crisis? Even though we know that we should remain positive, it's as if we've completely forgotten that. That is why God places certain people in our lives at certain times.

When I saw Jon pull in the driveway, I quickly hung up and got my shoes on. I couldn't get to the hospital fast enough. While driving to the hospital, my goal was to get there to save my baby. Even though I had not physically touched, smelled, or seen this miracle, he or she was mine. Jon had to stay home, as we didn't have anyone to watch our other children. This, unfortunately, was the reality of living far from family, but it's the life we chose willingly with his line of work. We've gotten used to it over the years, but it wasn't easy, especially in such moments.

As I pulled away, I didn't know how to feel. I tried to lean on God and trust that He held this situation. When I pray sometimes, I forget that His hand is holding the situation, even when it does not go as planned.

When I reached the hospital, attempting to describe why I was there was difficult, but that was the easy part. It was around nine o'clock in the evening at that point. I always find that the hospital starts to get quiet around that time, but that was not comforting to me; I wanted action and answers. Although they were working their way toward that, it felt like it was not enough. Of course, because I was on high alert, this situation was pressing for me. *Why aren't they hyped up like me?* I wondered. *This is serious. A life hangs in the balance.*

First, they wanted to perform some blood work to confirm HCG levels, which would help determine how far along I was and confirm the pregnancy. *Confirm the pregnancy?* I thought that was ridiculous. Did they think I was lying? Still, I knew that was the way these things were done, and they had protocol to follow. Obviously, I was not thinking clearly.

During the long wait for the blood work, my mind was focused on one thing: ultrasound. Why was it taking so long? That was surely the best way to see that all was normal.

The results finally came back. My HCG levels were low for the number of weeks I claimed to be pregnant. That was like a punch in the gut. What was happening? What did that mean? Why were they low?

Thankfully, the next step was the ultrasound, the doctors said, to confirm the pregnancy again. Now I was starting to get angry. *Of course I'm pregnant. I didn't make this up.* As I lay there on the hospital bed, cold and alone, I was scared of the results.

First, they attempted to do a regular ultrasound, but they couldn't see anything. They made statements like, "We don't see a pregnancy," and "There is nothing there."

I lay there, confused and broken.

Hope rose in me when the doctor decided to try a more invasive ultrasound using a tiny camera that could get closer to the womb. I thought, *Yes, exactly. My baby is just really small.* Again, the doctor looked in silence, but I remained hopeful. He wanted a second opinion. He didn't tell me anything before he left the room to get a colleague. I had to be positive; there was nothing left but to do that. I firmly believed he was getting a colleague to confirm the presence of my baby. *Protect my baby, touch my baby, show me my baby. Please, Lord*—this was the prayer continually racing in my mind.

Both doctors came in together and were very silent. The silence was killing me. Why did it have to be so quiet? I hated that it was the middle of the night, but I couldn't wait for the light of day. Once again, I remained still so they could look for my baby or "pregnancy" or "fetus," as they called it. That just boiled my blood. I wished they would call it what it was—*a baby, my baby*!

After what felt like hours of silence, they told me there was no fetus present. They even asked if I was really pregnant. Talk about insulting and being made to feel as if I'd lied. In hindsight, I am aware they had to ask those questions; everyone has a job to do.

"Yes, I'm pregnant. I have a pregnancy test at home that shows positive!" I told them. Following seemingly a million questions, something they said started to make sense. The amniotic sac was present, but no heartbeat was detected.

My heart shattered. I didn't cry right away, though, as I felt shocked and filled with disbelief. They told me to stay a while longer so that they could decide on the next steps. I couldn't fully comprehend what was happening or what the next steps would look like.

I was "lucky" it wasn't busy that night, so they allowed me to lie down in a hospital bed in the ER while I waited. Not a soul was in my room, and I'd never felt so alone. I yearned for Jon to be by my side, not to have someone to talk to but a presence, someone who loved me and who would hold my hand through this.

I never cried at the hospital because it didn't feel like a possibility. I had to stay strong—who was going to pick me up? That night, I did not feel God's presence. That is not what most people want to hear. They want to hear that God was with me every step of the way, holding and embracing me during an impossible time. Sorry, but this was raw life. No rainbows or unicorns here.

Can we look at my statement a little closer, though? The operative words are *I did not feel*. Just because we don't feel God's presence does not mean He is not there. Often, we push Him away in the pain that's too hard to deal with. Sometimes, it is so much easier to feel nothing than to feel everything. In that particular moment, it was far better to just lie there and be numb to it all.

In the wee hours of the morning, I was finally discharged. I would have to go for another ultrasound and another doctor's appointment, but at that time, I was sent home.

When I got home, I jumped right in bed, closed the curtains, and buried myself under the blankets. I found no joy that day or in the days that followed. I could hear my kids getting up, but Jon had control of that.

It was Halloween that day, and I had planned to take my two-year-old to an inside mall walk to collect candy. That broke me as well—the fact I was too broken to take him. There was no strength in me, and this went on for what felt like forever, especially for Jon, I'm sure. He was gracious to me and picked up the slack and took time off work. That allowed me to grieve and, hopefully, heal.

If you think about it, wasn't he also grieving? He told me that he was sure it was harder for me because I had that connection with the baby. I have no doubt that he was right, but I will forever be thankful to him for picking up the slack.

It was not over. More ultrasounds and doctor visits. At the doctor visit, someone finally explained what was happening. My body was not doing what it should have done, which was miscarry on its own. So I had to have a procedure to remove the pregnancy. The symbolism of my body not letting go was ironic to me. I was trying so hard to hold on to my baby. But the reality was that I needed this procedure for my own well-being and to heal properly.

When things become very dark in life, not much makes sense. In my mind, the baby clearly didn't want to go, and this completely ruined me, even though I was fully aware that's not how it works. Our bodies react a certain way, and sometimes we need help. I got that help, and I felt relieved when I woke from the surgery. The wait time before the surgery was approximately five days, and each day was filled with darkness and depression. I tortured myself, allowing my mind to go wherever it wanted.

We had to explain to our kids what their maman was going through. Jon surprised me by using a great analogy, one that even my two-year-old understood: sometimes, when you plant a flower, it does not always fully grow, or it fails to grow at all. My baby failed to grow—so simple yet so complex in the natural mind.

When I got home from my surgery, a certain weight was lifted from my shoulders. But just because I felt lighter didn't mean the spirit of depression stopped lingering. And then anger started to kick in. I was angry with two things: myself and God. Guilt is a powerful tactic. What if I had done something different? What did I do wrong? Should I have eaten differently or not eaten something in particular? Maybe it was last week's walk. I pushed myself too much. Did I forget to take my vitamins too many times? Not enough folic acid? The list went on and on.

But the reality is that these things happen, and it's not your fault. In a situation like this, you most likely will never get an explanation. You can drive yourself up the wall trying to think of a reason, and maybe you'll come up with a valid one, but you will never know.

I was so mad at God. This was the first time I'd felt that way toward Him. I believe that He is OK with our being angry with Him. It's better than walking away from Him completely. He knows that we are dealing with real human emotions. Jesus was here physical, as a human, and felt all the emotions we feel. Didn't He get frustrated and angry with the things He lived through. Certainly, He did, but He had far more control.

On Sunday when I went to church, my body was there, but my heart was not. I stood with my arms crossed as so many emotions—mainly anger—flowed through me. I love to worship, sing, and dance in the Lord's presence. Many of us connect with God through music. It helps us to enter into His presence.

On that Sunday, though, it was like I said to God, "Here I am, but don't expect me to be joyful about it." Some might say that at least I showed up, and they wouldn't be wrong, but a part of me will always wish I could have worshiped Him, even in that dark time. I was so upset that I couldn't understand how He had allowed this to happen.

Do you ever look back on your life and think you had all your ducks in a row? I chuckle a bit when I think of that analogy because I once saw a meme on Facebook that said, "I don't have ducks or a row. I have squirrels at a rave!" There have been many times in my parenting career when that best described how I felt.

When we decided to try having a baby after our miscarriage, I felt like my ducks were in a row. I had a job as a law clerk that I loved. My kids were all in school. The Lord had blessed us with a home that was perfect for our needs. We were finally living close to the church we attended, which was something we had prayed for. We were more than blessed; what more could a person ask for?

This time, though, I went into it differently. I was set on doing all the right things. Jon and I never had an issue with fertility; that was not the problem. When I made my mind up, it did not take long for us to get a positive pregnancy test. Approximately a month before, I had started to take prenatal vitamins. Healthy eating and getting lots of rest were also in the back of my mind as I entered this pregnancy.

I was scared, so like most humans, I found the things in life that I could control, and I was sure that would make a difference in the outcome—but I was still carrying guilt around with me.

I continued to work at my job for the kindest lawyer imaginable. Having already had three successful pregnancies, I knew what symptoms to look for. Our oldest son nearly killed me with nausea and dehydration. I was hospitalized because I couldn't eat or drink with him. Then our sweet daughter came along, and I was not nearly as sick, but the morning sickness, which is not limited to the morning, was still very present. I worked up to the end of the first trimester and felt ill but functional. Perhaps it's something to do with gender, as our youngest son also had me feeling very sick.

Thank the Lord, my mom came to visit in the first trimester of our third pregnancy. My days were made up of attempting to get dressed, lying on the couch, and hoping I'd be able to stomach some food. When I didn't feel significantly ill with this pregnancy, I started to worry that something was wrong, but I kept telling myself that all pregnancies are different. I thought it might have to do with being so busy with work and life that there was no time to feel the nausea.

Jon and I were both so excited when ultrasound day came around. I couldn't wait to see that little heartbeat on the monitor. On top of that, my ol' bean was visiting from Manitoba. What a great weekend it was going to be! I had planned to show her the ultrasound picture and share my joy.

As we waited for our turn, I managed to keep any negative thoughts out of my mind. Jon is a very positive person, so having him with me helped. This time, I was not alone, and for that, I was thankful. He had to take time off of work, but family has always come first for him.

As the technician placed the ultrasound wand on my abdomen, I began searching for the blinking light on the monitor. The technician moved from side to side and up and down but remained silent. She then asked, "How far along are you?"

Oh no! I thought. *Not that question!* I calmly told her and waited for a response. She then suggested that we perform the internal ultrasound. This was starting to feel all too familiar to me, but she tried to reassure me that sometimes the fetus is too small.

As she set up for the internal ultrasound, Jon reassured me that it would be OK. He's so full of joy all the time. Standing there, waiting, he said things like:

"Can't wait to see the heartbeat!"

"Can you believe we will have four kids?"

"How fun will it be to hold a newborn again"

The technician was so kind; she did her best to find my baby's heartbeat, but the thing that happened last time was occurring again, and I simply couldn't fathom it. Tears rolled down my face as I remained very silent. I wanted to get out of there as fast as humanly possible.

Jon listened to the instructions for what would come next—another surgery to remove the amniotic sac. In Ontario, we get so much snow that most doctors' offices require you to take your boots off before entering. As I bent down to pull my boots on, I broke. As a shy person, it goes against my nature to be loud, especially in a public setting, but this was out of my control. I broke down in disbelief that this was happening again.

Jon told me it was all right, and I'm sure he was not quite sure how to handle my emotions.

"No, it's not OK," I kept saying over and over again. "How is this OK? I've ruined everything. I failed. I'm broken. Something is wrong with me."

It was no longer about God; it was about me and the failure that I was. I'd done everything right!

I was raised in a home where fresh cookies, cakes, breads, squares, and any other mouth-watering bakery item was a common occurrence. As a result, I enjoy baking; it soothes my soul. If I'm having an off-day, baking muffins or cinnamon buns can be just the right pick-me-up. Baking cannot be compared to cooking. This is something I learned when talking to several friends on the subject. When you cook a meal, you can add a little of this and a little of that, perhaps even change the ingredients. There is much more freedom in cooking. When you bake a cake, you can experiment with flavors, but you must follow a recipe to get the right result. Add a little too much baking soda, and the cake might taste off. Forget to add an ingredient, and it could mean a flop! I followed the right recipe for the perfect cake, which is why I didn't understand why my cake didn't rise. I'd added the eggs, baking powder, flour, salt, milk, oil, and a whole lot of love with precision.

From that ultrasound, we were told to see our family doctor to discuss the next steps. At that appointment, I was given the choice to either take medication that would cause me to miscarry or to have a dilation and curettage. Our doctor did warn me, though, that the more D&Cs I underwent, the harder it might be for me to have a successful pregnancy.

Being in the moment, overwhelmed, hurt, and angry, I told him that it didn't matter because I was done trying. I didn't make this decision on my own; Jon agreed with me. There was only so much heartache we could take. We were already blessed with three children; perhaps that was what God wanted for us. I chose the surgery because I could not wrap my mind around taking something that would cause me to miscarry.

Funny—I was all about control before, but in that situation, I didn't want to have anything to do with it. If this was going to happen, it was not going to be by my hand. Please remember we all think differently, and there is no judgment here. I'm simply sharing what went on in my mind. I didn't want any recollection of this procedure. I thought it was best for me to just be done with it. It was easier for me to go to sleep and wake up with it behind me.

This time around, Jon was allowed to come with me for the procedure. We waited for what seemed like forever in the hallway before we were brought into the pre-op room. From there, we had to part ways when it was time for the procedure. The surgeon was so kind; she asked if a recent ultrasound had been done so we could be sure there really was no heartbeat. You have no idea how much that meant to me. This doctor was the first to really acknowledge that a "fetus" was alive and was a baby to me.

As I woke up to see Jon holding my hand, I knew that, in time, it would be OK.

Never underestimate the power of having someone by your side. There need not be any words said but simply the presence of another person in your corner. The presence of God is very similar at times. He may not send big signs, and maybe you are the only one who can feel Him.

When I think about the first miscarriage and how awful it felt to be alone, I realize that I might not have been upset only about the miscarriage. Deep within me, the anger mostly stemmed from one question: *Where were you, God?* I felt so alone. I didn't feel His presence. There will be dry seasons in our walks with God, where it is difficult to feel and see Him. Maybe that's the point, though. Are we still able to praise Him in the darkness and when He is quiet?

Thriving in dark and dry places is where we find our joy. Plants are much more resilient than you might realize. The perfect conditions that each plant needs to thrive are different, one from the other. A plant has the power to decide where and how much of its energy to disperse, depending on its environment. They may not be able to control their circumstances, but often, they can choose how to react. In fact, there is a process called *vernalization*, in which the plant will flower despite being exposed to a long period of cold. When the cold has passed, the plant will know when it's safe to flower, after guarding itself from the cold.

I have a plant that I've kept in my back room on a high shelf, away from natural light, and it has even been forgotten. I haven't watered it in over a month. I placed it there because it looked dead over a month ago, not a green leaf on it. But now, it is full of beautiful green leaves, after a month of dark and dry circumstances. Miraculously, it chose to thrive in its unfavorable circumstances. When it should have died, somehow, it found the strength to find joy. Like this plant and many others, you have the power to choose joy and bloom in the dark. God is still with you in the cold exposure, and soon, your time to flower will come.

Have you ever read the story of Job? If you haven't, I strongly urge you to do so—not because it will uplift you because Job had it rough. Job was very depressed and even seemed angry with God. But when you read farther, you'll learn about all of his losses and will quickly understand why he felt that way. Job must have wondered where God was. Did he ever doubt the presence of God? Nope. When he wondered where God was, he was referring to God in his own life. He knew there was a very mighty and wonderful God, and he continued to praise Him.

We have all felt like Job at one point or another, but James 1:2–3 says,

> My brethren, count it all joy when ye fall into divers temptations; Knowing this, that the trying of your faith worketh patience.

We need to hang on to God's joy through all our hardships and see a greater purpose. When we can't see that purpose, there is still a hope found in God, knowing He works all things together for our good.

These miscarriages were a pivotal time in my life, a time when joy was not within my reach. God puts us through hard times for the purpose of finding His joy. Through it all, I learned to find joy within the pain. I believe that these particular events were exactly for that. As I began to heal, I could feel my internal joy shift from the things this world could offer me to who God was for me. Although it seemed like a time when no joy was to be found, the problem was that it was dependent on my circumstances. I knew that if I wanted joy, I would have to choose to be filled with it.

We all muddle through difficult circumstances. It doesn't matter who we are, but the question is, where does our joy come from? From my heartache, I've been able to look at my circumstances differently and know from where my joy stems.

God can still be the goodness in our lives, even in the midst of the storms. When our joy is found in Him, our circumstances don't weigh us down because of the one thing that stays the same. We must choose to focus on God and find our joy wholly within Him. The "joy" of this world fades and is forever changing.

A few years later, I got to hold our fourth child in my arms right after she arrived. I was filled with an instant joy and thankfulness, but seconds later, she was pulled from my arms. I'd lost a significant amount of blood during childbirth, and the nurses were trying to get it under control. Jon and I locked eyes; no words were needed. This was his worst fear—losing his wife during childbirth.

Surprisingly, I found myself with an intense amount of peace and joy. The fear of losing my life did not have its grip on me. I was only thankful that I'd had a chance to hold and see our baby girl, Esmée. If it was my time to go, and meet my Creator, then I was OK with that idea. Clearly, I pulled through, but the peace and joy I felt within that uncertain circumstance is forever engraved in my heart and soul.

Now the God of hope fill you with all joy and peace
in believing, that ye may abound in hope, through
the power of the Holy Ghost. (Romans 15:13)

The joy with which God will fill you will provide you with
the hope you need to walk through dark waters. His joy remains
the same, no matter the day or time. When you are filled with His
joy, it will also freely flow from you so you can share it with others
around you.

Play the song "Joy" by For King and Country—one of my
favorite Christian bands—and I challenge you to choose joy! Healing
comes from allowing God's joy in your life, although you may not
feel it quite yet. This joy is not the absence of pain or heartache but
the ability to persevere through your tragedies.

1. What tragedies have shaken you and perhaps left you feeling empty and joyless?

2. Was there a time when you felt that God was not by your side? Can you look back with perspective and see Him in the chaos?

3. As a plant goes through dark and dry circumstances, you might feel that way too. Remember the plant will flourish after a long cold period, called vernalization. Use any hope within you, and write down what the joy of the Lord would look like in your life, as you decide to choose joy.

4. Turn on the song "Joy" from For King and Country, and pray that God will fill you with His joy. Enter into His presence, and let this joy consume your very being, forever changing who you are.

14

MOSAIC
MASTERPIECE

Before the pandemic hit, I had started taking pottery classes. As my youngest was then about eight years old, it seemed I'd have time for a new hobby. When the kids were infants and toddlers, it was difficult to embark on a new activity—it's not impossible, but more planning is required.

The idea of taking a piece of clay and shaping it into an object sounded fun and satisfying; it was an aspiration I'd had for years. I really wanted to learn to make mugs of different shapes and sizes—I love my cup of coffee. The idea of making beautiful mugs to drink my coffee from—what a wonderful idea! That fire was kindled to the next level when we vacationed in Prince Edward Island (PEI) one summer. It was inspiring to see the wide array of "makers" in that area. Everywhere we went, there were handmade items of fine quality. Many of the boutiques carried at least a couple of local branded mugs and cups, and all of them were unique in their own way. I practiced willpower while browsing these shops; it was hard to choose just two from the vast collections.

PEI gives off a creative vibe; you can't visit and leave uninspired. The beaches alone are out of this world—red ocean water hitting gigantic rocks that are surrounded by red sand. You might think that a person who has lived in British Columbia, as I have, would be used to the ocean, but it was another world in this province.

I'm constantly surprised by the beauty and magnitude of God's creation. The island is cottage country and has a permanent vacation atmosphere. When we returned from the best vacation we'd experienced in a long time, I was motivated and determined to try my hand at pottery, so one of the first things I did was enroll in a pottery class. In this class, I would get to use a pottery wheel to form my creation. I decided that I was going all in and was so excited to finally be giving this a try.

This particular pottery location radiated creativity as soon as I stepped inside. Flashes of color were all over the place, and there were many shelves displaying students' creations. I felt right in my element the minute I walked in the door. The first lesson did not disappoint; between various instructions, we used the wheel that same day. The instructor gave careful directions to facilitate the steep learning curve of handling the wheel and the clay at the same time. Apart from important detailed tips, I found that this skill would be learned over time, and with much practice. The instructor could voice the steps all she wanted, but the true results came from knowing how to feel your way by manipulating the clay.

As my foot slowly pressed down on the pedal and the clay glided through my hands, I felt at peace and soothed by this activity. Clay water splashed and hit my body, and I then understood the need for aprons. The soft, malleable clay slid every which way, depending on where I applied pressure. Several times, the clay would tilt more to one side, and it was my job to bring it back to the right position. I could understand how every piece of pottery was unique when I had a hand in creating them. No piece is the same as any other. Of course, a skilled potter can recreate a specific design, but there will be slight differences from the original. There is such a beautiful message in that idea. We are all created by the same God, but each of us is uniquely made.

I found the class to be much more difficult than I had imagined. Several times, I had to restart my creation. Flaws are all part of the pottery-making process, but there are times when the creation is simply too far gone. Then the best solution is to break it down and rebuild from scratch. I was thankful that I had the opportunity to rebuild when things were not going as planned. How much more difficult would it have been if, once I messed up, there was no point of return. It would be frustrating, and most people might even give up.

There is a story in Jeremiah that speaks to the idea that the Lord is the potter and has the ability to either rebuild, tear down, or destroy.

> Then I went down to the potter's house, and, behold, he wrought a work on the wheels. And the vessel that he made of clay was marred in the hand of the potter: so he made it again another vessel, as seemed good to the potter to make it. (Jeremiah 18:3–4)

God has the power to decide when something or someone needs to be reshaped or given a new beginning. This story is more than just an analogy about God being the potter. Jeremiah received this message from the Lord because the people, Judah, were doing evil in God's sight. Because of this, God had to make some difficult parenting decisions. He had good plans for them, but they were not behaving, which forced Him to rethink the initial plan. Later in this chapter in Jeremiah, God warns the people about the path they are choosing.

God wants to shape and mold us for His good plans, but ultimately, we decide to be teachable or not.

God, your Creator, held you in His hands, shaped you, and molded you perfectly into the vessel that He knew was good.

> But now, O LORD, thou art our father; we are the
> clay, and thou our potter; and we all are the work
> of thy hand. (Isaiah 64:8)

God knew that as we grew, He would have to reshape or even break us. This is a necessary process for spiritual growth and healing within our souls.

Jon has told me that when he was a child, he suffered through "growing pains." He grew so fast that the process caused leg pain in the night, which kept him awake, crying, at all hours of the night. It was a necessary evil for his growth but painful nonetheless.

Nothing in this world remains the same. The only thing that we can count on staying the same is God, as He is the same yesterday, today, and tomorrow. No doubt God puts us through difficult situations that will reshape who we are and help us grow spiritually.

The potter that is our God continues to spin the wheel for our good and perhaps for our healing. As he holds us and presses on the pedal, there will be times when He applies some pressure for redirection, all according to His good plan. We all go through situations that leave us wondering why God allowed that to happen. We believe we are on the right track; then, out of nowhere, something halts the process. The pressure He applies is usually to get us back on the right path or to help us grow. As we grow, we heal.

Breaking a bone is extremely painful, something to which Jon can attest. As a kid, he broke his tibia twice and broke a bone or two playing hockey, but the bones healed after the breaks. Unlike a bone, however, a broken individual usually comes out stronger on the other side. It is in the brokenness where we find true healing. We have to allow God to apply the pressure, and we must go with the flow while holding on to His promises with everything we have.

I can't tell you how many times I have been broken, disappointed, sad, and just plain confused. When we were living up north in Manitoba, Jon and I decided that we would become a foster family. We already had three kids, but we were in a community that needed foster families, and we had the desire, so it seemed like a no-brainer to us. We had the privilege of fostering a couple of babies for a short time. Then we were blessed with a long-term fostering opportunity for a little girl around age three. We were beyond ecstatic when the case worker told us there was potential for adoption. Jon and I had always had a heart to welcome another child into our home. We weren't naive about all the children looking for a home, and we believed that this could be an option for us.

The excitement ended quickly when her parents started to fight the idea of their daughter being adopted. Allegations were made against Jon and me that we couldn't ignore, and in the best interest of our children, we had to stop the process. I was crushed and broken.

Our family had quickly come to love the little girl and had incorporated her into our daily life. I treated her just like my other three children; in my heart, there was no difference. She had become one of my babies. I wanted to give her the absolute best. Several times, we made the trip down to Winnipeg, which was an eight-hour drive, so that she could get her proper dental care. I tucked her in at night with a hug and kiss on the cheek, telling her how much we loved her.

Did I understand why this was happening? Absolutely not! I felt broken and shattered about the situation. My heart ached not only because I felt like we'd lost a child but also for this young girl who would be tossed around from home to home. But if I was able to give that little girl just a little bit of love, then perhaps she could carry that with her. I'll never understand why that happened. I need to believe it was the plan. Isn't that what faith is—to believe in the unseen? That remains true for the things that we do not understand. We must believe that God knows what we don't.

Naomi from the book of Ruth echoes the principle of beauty in brokenness. She lost her husband and two sons at the same time. In those times, a widow would certainly face hard times, but her wonderful and stubborn daughter-in-law Ruth, who lost her husband too, stuck by Naomi through thick and thin, even to worshipping the God that Naomi loved, without knowing who this God was.

Ruth's mother-in-law was broken, but Naomi refused to stop seeing the beauty that could be. She had enough love and faith for both of them. Ruth ended up marrying Boaz and giving birth to a son named Obed. Obed was the father of Jesse, who was the father of David. Quite the lineage in which Naomi and Ruth had a hand, especially when they thought that it was all over for them. God had good plans for both of them, even though it did not feel like it at the time.

As life continued to throw curveballs at me, chips began to break off the vessel that is me. Miscarriages, depression, anxiety, loss, grief, and unworthiness all knocked big chunks off me. What once was a perfectly formed vessel slowly broke apart. I thought, *I can't be broken. Too many people are watching me. Little people are watching me, and they require a strong parental figure.*

But the thing is our little people will grow and go through trials. Life will break them, as it often does. Allowing others to see us when we're broken gives them the permission to break too. If we only show strength all the time, whether real or fake, our children will think that it is wrong to feel broken. We often ask God to hold us together, while He is telling us to let ourselves break. Superwoman, Superman, Ironman, Captain America, or Hulk are what we attempt to be when we were not meant to be that. God is that—and more—for us, if we allow Him.

As I grow older, my body can't take as much as it once could. I'm not old, but life sure can make me feel that way sometimes. I used to be able to go for days on end with little sleep; now, my body signals me when it's running low. My soul tells me the same as I keep taking the hits. When my soul is weary, my mind and body follow suit. How much more should I take before I surrender to being broken?

The thing is, God waits until we allow ourselves to be vulnerable. When we can do that, we open a new level in our spiritual walks and healing. Only as we allow ourselves to be broken wide open can we empty ourselves completely and allow room for a complete and new healing in our souls. When we hold on to our hurt, pain, and brokenness, we are not ready to receive His healing

As a vessel falls and breaks, we may think that it is over, but it's only the beginning of a beautiful healing journey. I believe there is a profound message in the story of the woman who anoints Jesus with the ointment of spikenard. The alabaster flask that held this very expensive perfume was also valuable. Alabaster is a hard stone that would have been difficult to break open. The woman would have to have been very intentional about breaking open the flask. Those who were present to witness her anoint Jesus with the ointment became upset with the woman. They were fully aware of the value of this ointment and knew it could have been sold for a lot of money.

Let's examine this woman's heart and intention concerning her actions. I've heard this story preached many times, but as I was writing this chapter, a new perspective touched my heart. As the woman broke the alabaster flask to pour the ointment on Jesus, I believe she saw the bigger picture. The ointment in the flask may have been valuable, but she knew that what Jesus had was priceless and far greater.

We may hold on to what we have inside. We may believe that we need to conserve the contents and are scared of what we will lose if we break from the inside out. But if we allow ourselves to break, Jesus can rebuild us in a way we never thought possible. What if all we need to do is allow ourselves to break so that Jesus can do exactly what He came to do? He came for the broken, not for the perfect.

As I continue down this bumpy and erratic path called life, I've learned that the healing is in the breaking. As I was writing this book, a new level of anxiety hit me. The daily struggle was very real as I tried to make it through every day. *Broken* is the perfect word to describe how I felt most days. I couldn't understand what was happening. I started this life as a brand-new, whole vessel, but with each passing day, I felt I was breaking, piece by piece. Would I ever be the same person I was years ago?

Then one morning, I came to a simple yet powerful revelation. The night before, I had struggled greatly with my anxiety. I had tossed and turned for hours, unable to fall asleep. It felt like slow torture. That next morning, I had several appointments for myself and for my children. The checkbox option "sick" was not on the list that day.. I had to be alive and alert.

I had set my alarm for earlier that morning so that I could have my Bible reading and devotion time. I had to force myself to get out of bed as the alarm went off. I felt like a shell of myself and wasn't sure how I would get through the day. I went to the only option on my list for help. As I entered into prayer, begging for God's help and filling Him in with all the details of my current state, I could feel myself being lifted up. I explained to God that without His divine strength, it felt impossible to walk through the day. I asked for *help*, as I believed, within my brokenness, that He could put me back together.

That day went flawlessly. I was on time for an appointment that I had thought I should have canceled—my daughter's dentist appointment was too close to mine, and it would have taken a miracle to make it on time. A miracle is exactly what I was given, among others that followed that same day. A simple prayer of help was answered in an extremely big way. To ask for help is to be vulnerable; it is knowing that we are broken and that the potter has the ability to piece us back together.

A mosaic is a picture or pattern that is made with small pieces of hard material. The pieces are placed beside each other to create a beautiful image or pattern. Many different types of materials can be used, such as seashells, glass, broken cup pieces, or stones—just about anything. With such an extraordinarily detailed piece of art, my eyes fly all over the place, taking in every intricate piece. No piece is the same; each is unique and broken in a different way.

My daughter Novalee recently started collecting beach glass and pebbles. As she was speaking with her aunt about her growing collection, her aunt suggested that Novalee create a mosaic when she had enough pieces. This might take some time, as she doesn't find beach glass every time she explores, but it's a wonderful goal to work toward.

Similar to a mosaic, God will piece us together into an even more beautiful creation. My daughter needs to be patient as she collects the pieces of beach glass to create a mosaic, and we need to apply this concept to our lives. We do not simply shatter in one fell swoop; it is a process that happens over time. With each hurtful and painful event, a few pieces may break off the vessel God has formed. But as we break and hand it over to Him, God will ever so gently create our mosaics. Through this vulnerability and brokenness, we will begin to feel whole and healed in our souls. The potter that is God shapes us on a continual basis, and our mosaic masterpieces are no different.

Our brokenness is the very thing that is needed to create a mosaic masterpiece. The song "Lay It Down" by Jordan St. Cyr says it well. He sings that we never think we will be the one to sink or be broken. But we can sing in the brokenness, knowing that God is our everything and that we may lay it down at His feet.

As you begin to lay down your broken pieces at Jesus's feet, you will be wholly healed within your soul. You can lay down the shame, unworthiness, guilt, hurt, pain, and insecurities for the greater purpose He has for you. This is life, and the world can be cruel, but there is beauty in your brokenness.

God knew that we would break in this world, but He also had a plan to beautify our broken pieces into a mosaic masterpiece. He is not scared of the broken us. I believe He'd like for us to embrace it. There is healing in acknowledging what we've been through and then allowing ourselves to let it go.

My husband, Jon, often says, "That sounds like a *you* problem." One day, I thought how appropriate that concept is for handing things over to God. This may sound harsh, but you need to place that broken piece at His feet and then say, "Well, God, this sounds like it is a *You* problem now!" I pray that you will be able to lay it all down and authorize Him to create a mosaic masterpiece within you.

1. Isaiah 64:8 tells us that we are the clay, and God is the potter. Has God shaped you lately? Have you experienced "growing pains" as He puts gentle pressure on you for your good? Write them down, and think about what God might be trying to tell you.

2. Have certain circumstances within your life caused you to feel shattered or broken?

3. Now that you have identified your brokenness, pray that God will slowly piece you together into the mosaic masterpiece that you are. How can you use your brokenness for good?

4. While you listen to the song "Lay It Down" by Jordan St. Cyr, let God take all the brokenness that you carry. Give it to Him, today and every day, so you can start walking in your healing.

15

DANCE IT OUT!

This is the last piece of the puzzle—the pièce de résistance. It's hard for me to believe that I'm writing the final chapter. Somehow, it felt like I would never get here. Then, at times, I knew that this entire book was within me; all I needed to do was flesh it out.

I'd like to thank you for reading my book. I've prayed, prayed, and prayed some more over this book. I have asked God for this book to be for His glory and that as people read my story, they will see themselves and find their healing, knowing that God wants that for them.

I have wonderful memories of doing puzzles with my family. My mom adores doing them with my kids. I have flashbacks of sitting around the big kitchen table with tea or coffee in hand, trying to put the pieces of the puzzle together—it requires much patience. It's an activity that not all people enjoy. There are those who find it mundane or more like work than a relaxing activity, but my kids and I thoroughly enjoy tackling a large puzzle together, especially on a rainy day or during the winter, when we don't feel like venturing outside.

Grab a "cuppa" of your favorite drink, grab a blanket, turn on some music, and maybe light a fire or a candle. Then, allow yourself

172

to drift into a world of relaxation, where all the worries of life seem far away. As you come close to finishing your puzzle, anticipation and excitement start to set in. You are almost there; soon the whole puzzle will be complete. But then, frustration sets in as you furiously search for the last few puzzle pieces. You have only a bit left to go, but you're not quite sure where all the pieces fit. You think it should be easy with so few pieces left, but perhaps you get tunnel vision. "Where is the last piece?" you ask yourself. "What will make this whole?"

This chapter is the last piece you need—the last piece I needed. I desperately searched for the thing that would heal me as a whole. Deep down inside, I knew that there was something still to learn in the process that God was walking me through. I just couldn't put my finger on it.

It's similar to when you start looking for something in the house and then you get sidetracked. The garbage needs to be emptied, the dishwasher requires unloading, and you also have that load of laundry to throw in the dryer. Once you are finished with all the tasks that sidetracked you, only then do you remember that you were looking for something. But what was it that you were looking for? How frustrating when you can't even recall what you were searching for.

As I wrote this book, God continued to heal me and show me things I didn't know I needed to know. When I started writing, I sensed within my soul that there was no rush, that slower would be better. I didn't completely understand why, and at times, I wondered if I was procrastinating. But the feeling that slow and steady was best kept hitting me strongly. I have gained great clarity as to why God wanted me to go slowly. He still had teachings, revelations, and healings for me to see. This book would not be complete if I had not listened to what He put on my heart.

In May, I started to feel that knock on my heart—the voice that God instills in us telling us that it is time. We are ready to go full speed ahead; it is time to get this done. Everything we have walked though is for exactly this moment. Every tear we've cried will be a testimony to someone.

Each time I felt the paralyzing pain of anxiety roll through and over me was for this very moment. The heartache I endured gave me strength exactly for this purpose—to share with you that there's a light and healing far greater than you could ever imagine. It is not just for those around you or for a select few whom God deems worthy. It is for you, me, our neighbors, our family and friends, and those living in a different country—people we don't even know. This is for everyone. *This is for you!*

Nothing could have prepared me for what happened in the month of May. As I've mentioned, Ladies Conference is my favorite yearly event. For the past two years, I've been blessed to travel and bunk with my "bean," Shaila, and a few other fabulous ladies. It's great to get away for three days sans kids and without a care in the world. The event provides all meals, and there are vendors of all sorts that stay open until midnight. The most delectable ice cream is provided on the second day. Last but not least, there is an array of activities available in the afternoon between services. Even with all the outstanding perks that Ladies Conference has to offer, that's not why I go every year. There is nothing like praising, worshipping, and praying with other women who have the same love for God that you have. The presence of God can't be denied within the four walls of the building and, most importantly, within us. At this event, I know that my soul will be renewed, refreshed, and spirit-filled to an incomparable level. And there is no doubt that I am not the only one who deeply needs this kind of experience every year.

I attend, expecting great things from God. It is a time when I can disconnect from all my responsibilities and allow God to do whatever He wants. There is no question in my mind that He will do something supernatural; the question is, with what will He blow me away this time? God can do anything, wherever and whenever He wants, and I expect miracles all the time.

The atmosphere that is created through collective worship and a deep need for God's presence allows for a unique heart of expectation. We gather for a weekend of much-needed fellowship, but a part of each of us whispers to God, "Lord, I need you so desperately. This is what I came for."

I came to this particular conference with a deep weight within my soul. Anxiety had latched its claws on me more than I had ever experienced. The fact that I wouldn't be home, sleeping in my own bed, caused me anxiety. Although excitement to attend the event was in my heart, the weight of what I'd been carrying for months also followed. This is why I knew that, no matter what, I needed to attend—because I knew that God was going to turn it around.

On our first night at the campgrounds, my friends and I had a nice meal planned with other ladies. Each of us picked up our supper and then met to eat together. Keeping it simple and fun was what this weekend was all about. As we began to eat, I could feel a stir within me—the anxiety was gripping me ever so slowly. I tried so hard to push it away with deep breathing, focusing on the conversation, and prayer in my mind, reminding myself who I had on my side. My attempts seemed futile. My breathing became more labored. I was getting hot, and nausea followed. Apparently, I hid it very well, as my ol' bean didn't notice that I was slowly suffering.

That is one of my superpowers—I can suffer from within but no one knows because of my skill of hiding how I feel. I say this is a superpower, but that is something I've worked on changing, as it is not good for me, mentally. Bottling up feelings will result in physical ailments. My mind was boggled as to why I was feeling this way. I was surrounded by ladies who loved me. This was a safe environment. I felt caught off guard.

The disappointment and shame that comes with anxiety is real. There is a feeling of weakness, of believing that we should be stronger, that our feelings are invalid. This was the last straw. Only four hours into this weekend, and already I was feeling defeated. Thankfully, I was with my ol' bean. When I told her how wretched

I felt, she insisted on coming up with a signal that we could use in the future.

It is refreshing when someone is supportive instead of shaming you. It lets you know that your presence is not a burden, as you believe it to be. That is why you hide your feelings—who wants to be a burden? If you hide your struggles, you may think, then everyone can go on with life as normal.

The support of my ol' bean means the world to me. I feel free to be human, with all my flaws, struggles, and pain.

As the weekend kicked off with an evening service, God showed up, as He does all the time. The first couple of services were filled with praise, worship, and some deep mourning. I was not the only one who poured out my heart to God. Remember that when you pour out, there is the potential to be refilled. I felt the need to bask in His presence and weep over all the things from the past year. In my heart, I knew He was working, but how? That was still the question at hand. Two services in, I wondered how God was going to lift the heaviness and heal my soul.

As the days progressed, I felt something in my soul that was different. There was a confidence that I had never felt before—confidence that I belonged in His kingdom, that I could shine my true personality, and that it was time to stop hiding. He had been working on this for months now, but it was instilled in me that weekend.

What does this have to do with healing? Trust me; it all fits together like the last pieces of a puzzle. God was leading me to what He was going to ask me to do that weekend.

As the last evening service came around, every lady was getting tired. Although this weekend was fun, we usually left exhausted. It was physically draining to be in a place of constant worship and prayer—and, often, weeping. But our souls felt like they were about to burst with the goodness of God.

The final evening was a mix of emotions; we all were ready for a good night's sleep, yet we could have stayed in that state of praise forever. As the worship team helped us enter into His presence through song, praise, and worship, we wept. So many of the ladies who surrounded us wept and allowed God to guide this service.

All that we should have wanted was for God to guide the service, not the other way around. His sweet presence fell upon us as we prayed for each other. My ol' bean was also fighting against anxiety but in different ways. We both needed a touch from God.

Our speaker that year was outstanding and spoke to all our hearts that weekend. Most importantly, God spoke to me that night on the level He was waiting for me to reach. After all the weeping, praying, and hearing of God's Word, we were called up to the altar. It was an altar call for anyone who needed something from God, so I marched up there, expecting to hear from Him. I went up to the altar, believing that I would lift my hands and cry out to him, which was exactly what happened—but then, something in me and the atmosphere shifted.

That's our God for you. You think He's going to the left, and then, suddenly, He swerves to the right. As my soul shifted gears, I felt God impress on me that it was time to dance. At first, I didn't understand what He meant or how this would heal me. But, as usual, He kept poking at my spirit. God impressed on me that I had wept enough and that it was now the time to dance. Furthermore, I needed to grab my ol' bean, and we were to "dance it out" together. He wanted us to hold hands and dance and leap in His presence. The healing was also in the ability to stop weeping and dance in His presence and to trust Him enough to leap, rejoice, and claim the good that was coming.

After a few minutes of the battle in my mind, I decided to tell my ol' bean what He wanted us to do. Without a thought, she agreed. We turned toward each other, clasped our hands together, looked in one another's eyes, and asked each other if we were ready. Were we ready? The answer was yes! In that moment, we started to leap as high as our feet would take us. We danced in the Lord and felt His presence free us. I felt like a child as we leaped that night, and maybe that was the beauty of it all. Scripture tells us to come to Him like children. I believe that is because of the freedom that children walk in and the faith they freely carry with them everywhere they go.

Anxiety is being bound by circumstances—your mind and other factors that you normally can't see or rationalize. It makes sense that God asked us to come to Him like children, jumping and leaping freely without any chains. As we leaped, I could feel myself change.

Have you ever watched small children dance? There usually is no form or reason to the way they move. They simply allow their bodies to move, doing whatever feels freeing as they express themselves. They throw their hands in the air, with feet flying here and there and head bobs and shoulder movement. One thing for sure: they do not care what anyone thinks of them as they dance. It's not about the "right moves," not with children. Their sole focus is moving freely.

As we leaped and danced in the Lord, I did not think about what we looked like. I was simply consumed with God's presence and goodness that allowed us to rejoice in Him that way. I felt, deep in my soul, that this was it—the very thing that God needed me to learn for healing.

Ecclesiastes 3:4 tells us that there is "A time to weep, and a time to laugh; a time to mourn, and a time to dance." I cannot tell you how profoundly I feel this to be true in my soul. There *is* a season for everything, even in our healing. We know that it's OK and healthy to cry, especially when we go through something hard. It is essential for us to express and acknowledge how we are feeling. Tears are sometimes the only way we can express ourselves; words don't seem like enough at times. So we weep and then we weep some more, but then we can get stuck in that phase and don't know how to get ourselves out. We usually want nothing more than to be freed from that phase. Getting stuck in our head or in this weeping stage prohibits us from moving on to the plans the Lord has for us.

Dancing in the Lord can free our minds from the things that would otherwise stop us from receiving what God has for us. Several studies have proven that dancing and singing reduce stress levels and increase the hormone serotonin. Serotonin is also known as the "happy hormone" or "feel good" chemical. This hormone plays several roles in our bodies, one of them being our mood. Have you ever tried to dance your heart out while you are stressed? You would need to physically push yourself, as your body does not enter into dance freely when stressed. When you get past this, however, the feeling of stress or anxiety fades away.

Perhaps we are to dance in the Lord to enter into His presence on an even more freeing level. We should let go of our stress, worries, grief, depression, and anxiety and lay them down at His feet. We allow Him to work in our situations when we no longer show inhibition. Think about this: when you try to enter into His presence, your heart must be open completely.

> Thou hast turned for me my mourning into dancing: thou hast put off my sackcloth, and girded me with gladness; To the end that my glory may sing praise to thee, and not be silent. O Lord my God, I will give thanks unto thee for ever. (Psalm 30:11–12)

I've mentioned that the Lord gave me confidence that weekend. I believe He filled me with confidence so that I would have the boldness to dance and praise freely in His presence. He knew I would need His confidence in order to reach the new level of boldness and healing He had for me. Remember that confidence from God is not the same as natural confidence. The type of confidence we receive from God is necessary for the walk on which He wishes to lead us. It allows us to know that we are worthy of His love and can claim healings, callings, and the life He has already purposed for us.

In 2 Samuel, we read that King David danced freely before the Lord. Not only did he dance freely, but he danced with all his might.

> And David danced before the Lord with all his
> might. And David was wearing a linen ephod. (2
> Samuel 6:14)

A *linen ephod* is considered a "holy garment." This detail must
have been included in the scripture for a purpose. In Exodus, we find
that the Lord commanded that the *linen ephod* be made and used
as a priestly garment. It was important that not just any old piece
of clothing was worn when someone came before the Lord. I found
it interesting that the above scripture specifies that David wore a
linen ephod. It signifies that David was not dancing just to dance.
He knew that this was a holy, sacred moment before the Lord and
that it should be treated as such.

We are to treat our dance in the same way that David did when
he brought back the ark of the covenant. Furthermore, David was
not putting on a performance; his dance was solely for the Lord. We
see this when his wife, Michal, got upset at him for the way David
danced before the Lord. David knew for whom he was dancing, and
that remained the only thing that mattered in his heart.

When you come before the Lord, you need to have the same
heart as David had. This is a moment between you and God only;
everything else around you is irrelevant. When you are able to enter
into that special moment and allow for His Spirit to take the lead,
then you are forever changed.

I've learned the importance of dancing it out every single day.
When we dance it out every day, God's mercies, healing, purpose,
and strength are set upon our souls and hearts. To truly dance it
out, we need to let it all go, forget about ourselves, and solely focus
on what God is to us. "Dancing it out" may not be literally dancing
every day but entering into His freedom, even when things don't look
or feel good. It is saying to God that no matter the circumstance, we
choose to worship wholeheartedly and without inhibition because
we know who our Savior is.

As I end this book that has long been within my heart and soul, I'd like you to listen to "I Thank God" by Maverick City Music. This is a powerful, purpose-filled song about the promise that God has for you. The chorus tells us that we are to thank the Master, for the gift of freedom He gives us. Through picking us up, healing us, and placing us on a firm foundation. Because of this we are forever changed and free, and will never be the same!

Before the chorus, the song sings of wandering in the night and having a weary soul. But then you meet a man you didn't know, and you're not alone. No matter what you're going through, the healing you may need today, or the darkness that encompasses your soul, there is an answer. Be brave enough to dance it out every single day, knowing who your master is, and allow Him to heal your heart and soul.

As you dance with Him, the cloud (your situation or problem) will begin to lift. Your daily healing is in knowing who holds it all and who makes you whole. The song repeats the phrase "get up out of that grave" several times. Although it's difficult, this is where your true healing lies—having the ability to get up and hold on to the freedom He has given you, knowing He has already overcome the world. With this promise in your mind, body, and soul, you can stand firm in your daily healing that makes you whole. Get a firm grip on your "sunrise," and don't let it slip between your fingers.

This perpetual healing is God-given and meant for you and me. It is the freedom to break the chains that this world wraps around us. As the ebb and flow of the tide continually changes, we adapt to surfing the waves. The waves that would have us sinking and gasping for air become exactly what our souls require. We learn to dance with the waves, following the flow and embracing the healing within the pain. We know who controls the dancing waves that we fear, and our wholeness comes from leaping with joy because of who He is. So now, dance it out!

1. Do you wholeheartedly believe that God wants to heal you daily? This question requires you to be honest with yourself.

2. Enter into prayer today, asking God to instill His confidence within you. This confidence will allow you to go to an entirely new level with Him.

3. Read Ecclesiastes 3:4 again. Which time does God have you walking through right now? Is it time for you to move on?

4. Do you know the next step that God is asking from you? If not, pray that He will show you. Read His Word for understanding. If you know, pray that He will guide and give you strength to take the next step(s).

5. Which waves in your life make you feel like you're sinking? Which daily tactics that you learned from this book can you use to dance with the waves instead?

6. Turn up the volume on "I Thank God" by Maverick City Music, and enter into a state of worship and dance. This is a sacred moment between you and God, just as David had in 2 Samuel. Open your heart, and let God work within you!

Manufactured by Amazon.ca
Bolton, ON